GENETICALLY ALTERED FOODS AND YOUR HEALTH

Ken Roseboro
Thomas Hirsch, Series Editor

Basic Health
PUBLICATIONS, INC.

The information contained in this book is based upon the research and personal and professional experiences of the author. It is not intended as a substitute for consulting with your physician or other healthcare provider. Any attempt to diagnose and treat an illness should be done under the direction of a healthcare professional.

The publisher does not advocate the use of any particular healthcare protocol but believes the information in this book should be available to the public. The publisher and author are not responsible for any adverse effects or consequences resulting from the use of the suggestions, preparations, or procedures discussed in this book. Should the reader have any questions concerning the appropriateness of any procedures or preparations mentioned, the author and the publisher strongly suggest consulting a professional healthcare advisor.

Series Editor: Thomas Hirsch • Typesetter: Gary A. Rosenberg
Series Cover Designer: Mike Stromberg

Basic Health Publications, Inc.
8200 Boulevard East • North Bergen, NJ 07047 • 1-800-575-8890

Library of Congress Cataloging-in-Publication Data

Roseboro, Ken, 1954–
    Genetically altered foods and your health : food at risk / Ken
Roseboro.—1st ed.
      p. cm.
    Includes bibliographical references and index.
    ISBN 1-59120-059-8
  1. Genetically modified foods—Toxicology—Popular works. I. Title.

  RA1258.R67 2004
  615.9'54—dc22

                                                            2004002389

Printed in the United States of America

10   9   8   7   6   5   4   3   2   1

CONTENTS

EDITOR'S NOTE

Dear Reader:

Welcome to the *Basic Earth Guide* series! As you know, the natural world is becoming degraded at an alarming rate. Hardly a day passes without a new headline about the effects of global warming, species loss, and other distressing environmental news. Incredibly, during every second of every day, more than an acre of the world's precious and irreplaceable rain forests is being lost. The depletion of beneficial oxygen-producing plants, which are part of the rain forest's ecosystem, makes us vulnerable to the 6,000 metric tons (13,230,000 pounds) of carbon dioxide emitted into the atmosphere each year. The subtraction of oxygen and the addition of carbon dioxide adversely affects everyone's health and quality of life. This example is but one of a number of environmental problems that beset us. Residues of toxic pollutants, ranging from pesticides in our food; chemicals in our homes such as cleaning agents, sealants, solvents, formaldehyde, and lead-contaminated paint; gas leakages from cookstoves; outgassings from plastics; fragrances in consumer products; to a host of other volatile substances, both indoors and outdoors, affect our health. Over time, chronic exposure to these substances compromise our immune system and contribute to various illnesses and health problems. Some experts caution that we have *only one generation of time* to reverse conditions in our polluted environment, or we shall experience *irreversible damage.* Many people feel that the problems are on such a vast scale, are so complex and overwhelming, that individual efforts are futile. They are wrong.

The *Basic Earth Guide* series demonstrates that you, as an individual, can take meaningful action. Each *Basic Earth Guide* sets forth a group of ecological problems you face daily, and provides alternative, environmentally sound, practical solutions. Each *Basic Earth Guide* provides the best researched ideas and up-to-date information to help you make ecologically sounder decisions in your day-to-day living. The *Guides* are written simply and lucidly for easy comprehension. Among topics covered are renewable energy, 'green' building and retrofitting, home care and maintenance, personal care products, and ecological lifestyles.

We hope that, as a reader of *Basic Earth Guides,* you will become better informed and motivated to improve the environmental quality of your life, as well as the lives of those around you. There *can* be a new world out there! We thank you for allowing us to introduce it to you.

Green regards,
Thomas Hirsch, series editor

P.S. Do let us know of additional subjects that interest you for us to consider as topics for future *Basic Earth Guides.* You can reach us at ngoldfind@basichealthpub.com.

INTRODUCTION

*"At the agricultural level, the food industry is heading
in two opposite directions. On the one hand there is the
organic movement. The other side is biotechnology."*

—Bob Swientek, editor in chief,
Prepared Foods magazine

A walk through the supermarket in America today
won't reveal anything out of the ordinary, just the
usual rows of familiar packaged foods—cereals, salad
dressings, canned goods, soft drinks, snack foods, candies,
and more—a cornucopia of processed foods. One sees all
the recognized brands. Everything looks familiar, appe-
tizing, and reassuring, the same as it's always been, right?

Not quite. A closer, microscopic look reveals some-
thing new and unfamiliar, a fundamental revolution in
how foods are made, a technology that some say makes
every consumer a guinea pig in a massive feeding experiment. The technology is genetic engineering, also known
as biotechnology, and those familiar foods now contain
ingredients from plants whose genetic makeup has been
altered. Scientists have taken genes, the blueprints for all
living things, from living organisms such as bacteria and

viruses and forcibly inserted them into corn, soybeans, and other food plants. Americans eat foods containing ingredients derived from these novel plants every day. The plants contain genes, for example, from a bacterium that thrives in herbicide waste ponds and from a powerful virus.

There is no mention of this change on food labels. The government doesn't require such labels, and food companies fear they would become a skull and crossbones to scare consumers away from their familiar brands. As a result, most consumers are unaware of the radical change to their foods.

Meanwhile, in the same average supermarket, a small but increasing number of foods are appearing that carry a label—a round green and white seal that reads "USDA Organic." These organic foods have been produced without chemical pesticides and fertilizers—and without genetic engineering.

Crisis in Agriculture

These two trends, genetic engineering and organic food production, are competing to win the favor of American consumers. Moreover, biotechnology and organic, two radically different food production systems, are viewed by many agricultural "experts" as the best solutions to the escalating crisis caused by industrial agriculture with its over-reliance on chemical pesticides, petroleum-based fertilizers, and single crop "monocultures" of corn and soybeans.

Industrial farming methods have increased crop yields, but at a great cost to human health, wildlife, and the environment. Water sources are polluted with pesticides and nitrogen fertilizers. Pesticide residues represent an increasing health threat, especially to children. Nearly one-third of the world's arable land has been lost to erosion due to industrial farming practices. Writing about the crisis in 1997, Fred Kirschenmann, director of the Leopold Center for Sustainable Agriculture, stated, "We have now reached a point where we need to make some radical course corrections if we want to survive beyond the next century with any kind of quality of life."

Food Fight

Proponents of genetic engineering and organic agriculture each claim their respective methods will make agriculture more sustainable. The two approaches are polar opposites. Genetic engineering is a new technology; organic agriculture is based on methods that have evolved over thousands of years. Genetically altered foods are controversial, sparking protests among consumers, farmers, and environmentalists worldwide. No one protests the production of organic foods. While the organic system views agriculture from a wide angle lens encompassing soil, plants, human beings, environment, and society, biotechnology views it from a microscopic focus on genes. On a larger scale, biotech farming favors centralized control over the food supply by a few multinational corporations; organic farming fosters localized food networks such as farmers' markets, community supported agriculture, and urban gardens.

Both systems share rapid growth. Acreage planted with genetically engineered crops in the United States increased from 2 million in 1996 to more than 96 million in 2002. In terms of money, government support, corporate influence, and crop acreage, biotech farming dominates. However, organic foods possess one critical advantage: consumer acceptance. The demand for organic food has increased 20 percent each year since 1990, making it the fastest-growing food category. There is no demand for genetically altered foods. In fact, many consumers try to avoid them.

In the food fight between biotech and organic, only one system may ultimately prevail. The stakes are high, with the future of food as well as human health and the environment hanging in the balance. Time will tell which method proves the most successful and beneficial to the world.

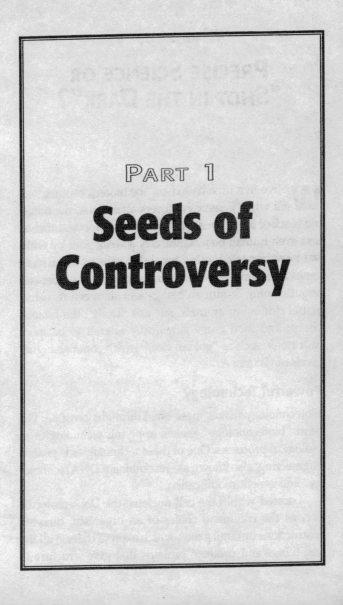

PART 1
Seeds of Controversy

Chapter 1

PRECISE SCIENCE OR "SHOT IN THE DARK"?

We live in a time hailed as "the biotech century," an era when genetic engineers alter DNA, the building block of life, to create new medicines, foods, animals, and even human beings. Scarcely a week goes by without news reports touting breakthroughs in identifying genes considered responsible for certain diseases; debates about cloning of human beings and stem cell research; actual cloning of animals, such as "Dolly" the famous sheep; and food crops genetically altered to be more nutritious, such as "golden rice," which contains higher levels of vitamin A.

Powerful Technology

Biotechnology makes these breakthroughs possible. The term "biotechnology" means applying technologies to biological processes. One of these technologies is genetic engineering, also known as "recombinant DNA technology" and genetic modification.

Located within the cell nucleus, the DNA molecule acts as the command center of an organism, carrying instructions through genes, which express traits in all living things and produce proteins that give structure to cells and direct their activities. Like pearls on a string, each gene occupies its own place in the DNA.

In genetic engineering of plants, molecular biologists remove one or more genes from the DNA of other organisms and "recombine" them into the DNA of the plant they want to alter. By adding these new genes, genetic engineers hope the plant will express the traits associated with the genes. For example, genetic engineers have transferred genes from a bacterium known as *Bacillus thuringiensis* or Bt into the DNA of corn. Bt genes express a protein that kills an insect, the corn borer, and transferring the genes, allows the corn to produce its own pesticide.

Genetic engineering has been described as one of the most powerful technologies ever developed because it breaks down nature's genetic barriers, allowing transfers of genes between microorganisms, plants, animals, and human beings. For example, genetic engineers have inserted genes from human beings into pigs to create animals with less fat. Genes from a flounder were spliced into the DNA of tomatoes to protect the fruit from frost damage. Such radical gene transfers could never happen in nature. For the first time in history, scientists can change the genetic makeup of all living beings.

Gene Guns and Bacterial Invaders

To create Bt corn, genetic engineers first isolate and remove the desired gene segment from the DNA of the Bt bacterium. Next, they assemble a sequence or "package" of genes needed to ensure that the gene from the bacterium works in the corn's DNA. One of these genes is called a "promoter," which "turns on" the new gene to express the desired trait. The promoter comes from a powerful virus called the Cauliflower Mosaic Virus. Another gene added to the package is an antibiotic resistant marker gene that acts like a flag to identify which corn cells have assimilated the gene package after it is transferred. Finally, a "terminator" gene is added to "turn off" the new gene.

Transferring the gene package into corn cells requires powerful methods, and genetic engineers have developed two that accomplish the task. The first is a "gene gun" that literally blasts the genes, shotgun like, through the cell walls. The second method uses a bacterium that invades a cell with the foreign genes. These invasive methods allow genetic engineers to break nature's genetic boundaries.

After gene transfer, the genes will attach to the corn genes at different points in the DNA. This random placement occurs because genetic engineers have no control over where the genes go.

To identify which genes have been accepted by the corn cells, scientists will add an antibiotic that will kill all cells except those with the marker gene, which is antibiotic resistant.

The transformed cells will develop into mature corn plants that will contain the pest-killing bacterium genes in every cell. Plant breeders will grow the plants over many generations to ensure the engineered trait is stable and continues to be expressed as desired.

Sculpture through the Window?

Proponents of genetic engineering claim their technology, as described on the Internet website of the Biotechnology Industry Organization, is "specific, precise, and predictable." They say it is precise because one or a few specific genes are transferred, unlike conventional crossbreeding of plants, which can involve the transfer of thousands of genes. Some scientists disagree about this precision. "When you insert a gene into a DNA using genetic modification, you have no idea where the gene goes, it's absolutely a shot in the dark," says John Fagan, chief scientific officer at Genetic ID, a laboratory that tests foods for genetically engineered ingredients.

According to one scientist, the process of inserting genes into the DNA of a cell is analogous to an artist who, in the hopes of having a sculpture exhibited in a museum, decides to bypass the usual channels required for exhibition and hurls the sculpture through the window. Clearly the artist doesn't know where the piece will land; it could roll under a table, smash into a wall, or even destroy another work of art. In the same way, genetic engineers have no idea where their inserted genes will "land" and what effects they will create on the genes of the host DNA. The foreign genes may be assimilated by the host genes and express the desired trait or they could cause mutations to the host genes, resulting in stunted, deformed plants or the creation of toxins or allergens.

"Genetic engineering is precise in terms of what gene goes in and what sequences are being added," says Margaret Mellon, a molecular biologist and director of the food and environment program at the Union of Concerned Scientists. "What we don't know is where the genes go relative to other genes, and how those genes will affect a very complicated system. We also don't know how these new plants will behave in an ecosystem. All this is very hard to predict."

As an example, in the early 1990s German researchers inserted a foreign gene into white petunia plants, which they predicted would turn the flowers red. They were surprised to find that some flowers turned red but then faded in color, others turned completely white, and others showed a mixture of red and white.

Because of this unpredictability, genetic engineers must grow and test hundreds or thousands of plants to find ones where the inserted genes work properly. It is estimated that only one in 10,000 gene transfers will succeed.

While engineering implies precision, genetic engineering involves complex biological processes that are often beyond human understanding and control.

GE Foods on the Market

In the early 1990s genetically engineered (GE) food products and crops began to enter the food supply. The first GE food product was chymosin, a substitute for an essential enzyme used to make cheese. This arrived on the market in 1990 and is now used to make more than half of all cheese produced in the United States.

In 1993 Monsanto Company, the leading producer of GE crops, introduced a GE product called "recombinant bovine growth hormone" (rBGH) that is injected into dairy cows to increase milk production. The U.S. Food and Drug Administration (FDA) approved rBGH, whose trade name is Posilac Bovine Somatotropin (BST), for sale in 1994. Introduction of rBGH caused the first major GE food controversy. Consumer activists claimed that milk from cows injected with rBGH contains high levels of Insulin growth factor-1 (IGF-1), which is considered a potent tumor promoter. Today, an estimated twenty to thirty percent of dairy cows in the United States receive injections of rBGH.

In 1994 the FDA approved the first whole GE food, the Flavr Savr tomato. The GE tomato was the creation of a U.S. company, Calgene, which engineered the tomato to increase its vine and shelf life by 90 percent. However, the GE tomato proved too costly to produce and was pulled from the market.

Roundup Ready

In 1996 Monsanto introduced what has become the most widely grown GE crop. Roundup Ready soybeans, which have been genetically engineered to make them resistant to sprays of Roundup herbicide, are Monsanto's best-selling product. The GE soybean plants are "ready" to be doused with Roundup and survive, while the weeds growing nearby die. The plants possess this unique ability thanks to a gene inserted from a bacterium that Monsanto's scientists found thriving in a chemical waste pond near one of the company's Roundup production plants. Monsanto also sells Roundup Ready corn, cotton, and canola, a plant used to make feed and cooking oil, and plans to introduce wheat, turf grass, and other Roundup Ready crops if consumers will accept them.

What GE Foods Are You Eating?

The FDA has approved more than fifty GE crops for the United States' food supply, including:

- Corn (15 varieties)
- Tomato (6 varieties)
- Cotton (5 varieties)
- Oilseed Rape (5 varieties)
- Canola (5 varieties)
- Soybean (3 varieties)
- Potato (4 varieties)

- Sugar Beet (2 varieties)
- Squash (2 varieties)
- Cantaloupe
- Rice
- Flax
- Raddicchio
- Papaya

Of these crops, only corn, soybeans, cotton, and canola are widely grown. Many of the other crops are either no longer sold due to market rejection, such as potato, sugar beet, flax, and tomato, or have never been commercially grown, such as rice. GE tobacco is grown, and is used to make Quest cigarettes.

However, GE field crops, such as corn, soybeans, cotton, and canola, maintain a dominant position in North American agriculture. More than eighty percent of soybeans grown in the United States are transgenic, GE cotton is grown on more than 70 percent of cotton fields, and GE corn is grown on about 35 percent of corn acreage. In Canada, GE canola accounts for more than 60 percent of the total crop.

Seventy Percent of Foods Contain GE Ingredients

GE crops now being grown are known as "first generation" genetically engineered crops. These crops aim to benefit farmers through insect resistance, as with Bt corn, or herbicide tolerance, as with Roundup Ready crops. Researchers at biotechnology companies and universities worldwide are now developing second and third generation GE food crops that aim to benefit consumers. These crops, which include grains, vegetables, and fruits, are being genetically engineered to enhance nutrition and even produce pharmaceutical drugs and vaccines.

An estimated 60 to 75 percent of processed foods found in retail food stores and restaurants contain ingredients that come from GE crops, particularly corn, soybean, and cotton. In the United States, corn and soybeans are processed into a wide range of food ingredients and vitamins found in many processed foods. Cotton seeds are processed into oil, which is also found in many foods.

Global GE crop acreage has increased from 4 million acres in 1996 to more than 167 million acres in 2003. The United States grows nearly 70 percent with more than 100 million acres. The other leading GE crop producing nations are Argentina, Canada, and China, which produces GE cotton. Other nations that grow GE crops include Australia, Columbia, Honduras, India, Indonesia, Romania and South Africa.

Backlash in Europe

Europe has shown the most resistance to GE crops. The introduction of GE crops in Europe coincided with the "Mad Cow" disease food scare in Great Britain in the late 1990s. In this tragic incident, cows given feed containing animal parts contracted a fatal brain-deteriorating disease, known as bovine spongiform encephalopathy (BSE). People who ate meat from the diseased animals contracted a similar disease, which caused more than 100 deaths. Mad Cow disease was then concealed from the public by the British government.

The scare caused Europeans to distrust government regulators and led to a huge consumer backlash against GE foods when they reached Europe in 1996. The British press dubbed GE foods "Frankenfoods" and protesters dressed in white sanitary suits ripped GE crops from test fields. In addition to safety concerns, Europeans, who valued their time-honored food traditions, did not accept the high-tech GE foods. Monsanto angered European consumers further when they tried to "educate" them about the value of GE crops.

As a result, the European Union's (EU) policy toward GE foods has been guided by the "precautionary principle," which states that the biotechnology industry must prove the safety of GE foods. The EU has established strict laws to label and trace GE foods and has blocked approvals of new GE crops since 1998. As of January 2004, the moratorium is still in effect.

The EU's policies have angered the United States, which is the leader in GE crop production, and in 2003 the United States filed a suit with the World Trade Organization in an attempt to end the moratorium.

Chapter 2

THE PROMISES AND PERILS OF GENETICALLY ENGINEERED FOODS

"We are at a stage in history when respect for the unfathomed natural order should override the unreliable ambitions of an already privileged and inordinately powerful minority of humans."

—Peter Willis, Ph.D., theoretical biologist in the department of physics, the University of Auckland, New Zealand (from an article in the *Canberra Times*, May 16, 2002)

Genetic engineering allows molecular biologists to take genes from one organism, and cross kingdom, phyla, and species, to insert them into another. To take genes from beta-carotene enzymes and insert them into rice to increase levels of vitamin A. To insert a gene from a petunia plant into a tomato to increase the production of antioxidants. To extract human genes and insert them into cows to produce human antibodies. With such infinite combinations possible, it is no wonder that many see great potential in the technology.

Horse and Automobile

While touting genetic engineering as a new and revolutionary technology, proponents also say it is simply an extension of traditional plant breeding. They claim it is faster, more precise, and accurate because it involves transferring just one or a few genes, while traditional breeding requires introducing hundreds of thousands of genes.

Some scientists disagree, stating that genetic engineering is radically different from conventional plant breeding. "It's like saying the automobile is an extension of a horse," says Philip Regal, professor in the department of ecology, evolution, and behavior in the College of Biological Sciences, University of Minnesota. "Genetic engineering is a powerful technique and a whole new area. It's not realistic to put them in the same category."

While genetic engineering allows transfers of genes from different plant and animal kingdoms and species, traditional plant breeding is restricted by natural genetic boundaries. Breeders must work within nature's laws to create new plants from the same or closely related species. For example, corn has evolved over thousands of years, and plant breeders have cross-bred many varieties to improve yields and quality. Genetic engineers, on the other hand, break down nature's genetic boundaries by forcibly inserting genes from an insect-killing bacterium and a virus into corn. Traditional plant breeders could never create potatoes with jellyfish genes, as genetic engineers have done.

"With traditional breeding, we have parameters, we know what is likely to turn up," says Margaret Mellon of the Union of Concerned Scientists. "With genetic engineering we don't know because it so new."

GE Promises

Proponents of genetic engineering promise an abundant harvest of benefits for mankind. They say GE crops will increase yields, reduce the need for agricultural chemicals, tolerate difficult growing conditions, and resist pests and disease. GE crops will create more nutritious foods, produce life-saving drugs and vaccines more economically, and help feed a growing world population. Proponents say that, while GE foods are new, they are "substantially equivalent" to conventional foods and pose no unique risks to human health or the environment. In fact, some say they are even safer than conventional foods.

Critics compare the promises of biotechnology with those of DDT when it was first introduced in the 1940s. The insecticide was hailed as a great breakthrough that would eradicate pests and lead to increased food production. Magazine ads claimed, "DDT is good for me" to emphasize its perceived safety for humans and animals. However, as time passed the negative effects of DDT surfaced as insects developed resistance and wildlife died from exposure. The use of DDT in the United States was banned in 1973.

Lower Yields

Do GE crops increase yields? Several studies indicate that GE soybeans yield less than conventional varieties. A study conducted at the University of Nebraska and published in the *Journal of Agronomy* found that GE soybeans yielded five to ten percent less than conventionally grown soybeans. Charles Benbrook, an agricultural economist and former executive of the board on agriculture at the National Academy of Sciences, found the same yield drag percentages when he analyzed field trial results comparing the performance of GE and conventional soybeans in Illinois, Minnesota, and Nebraska during the 1999 and 2000 growing seasons. A 2001 study of Iowa farms conducted by Iowa State University found that GE soybeans yielded 43.4 bushels per acre while conventional soybeans yielded 45 bushels per acre. Moreover, Iowa State University extension economist, Michael Duffy, concluded that farmers who plant GE corn and soybeans reap no greater financial gains than farmers who grow conventional crops.

Fewer Chemicals

Biotechnology proponents say GE crops allow farmers to reduce usage of environmentally damaging pesticides. For example, they say herbicide-resistant crops such as Roundup Ready soybeans allow farmers to use fewer types of herbicides and reduce the number of applications needed. Proponents claim Bt crops, particularly cotton, saved about 264,000 gallons of insecticide applications in the United States between 1998 and 2002. They also say GE herbicide-resistant crops have reduced the need to till or plow the soil to control weeds, which minimizes soil erosion.

Research by Benbrook refutes the claim about reduced pesticide usage. Analyzing USDA data, Benbrook found that Roundup Ready GE soybeans increased herbicide use by 70 million pounds from 1996 to 2003. Farmers planting GE Bt corn and cotton decreased insecticide use by a modest amount. Overall, total pesticide use has increased by 50 million pounds since the introduction of GE crops.

One organic farmer says that more herbicides are used with Roundup Ready cotton. "The more GE crops that are grown, the more spraying is done," says Terry Pepper, manager of the Texas Organic Cotton Marketing Cooperative, the largest producer of organic cotton in the United States. Pepper once lost a crop of organic oats due to drift from a crop duster spraying Roundup herbicide on a nearby field of Roundup Ready cotton.

Over-reliance on Roundup herbicide could spell doom for Roundup Ready crops. Weeds are becoming resistant to the Roundup herbicide and the lessening of its effectiveness weakens the rationale for Roundup Ready crops. This is an example of biotechnology's shortsightedness failing to account for nature's infinite adaptability.

Feed the World

Proponents say GE crops are needed to feed a world population that will increase to 10 billion by 2050. But, according to the United Nations Food and Agriculture Organization (FAO), enough food is grown worldwide to provide 4.3 pounds of food per person per day. Despite this, 800 million people worldwide go hungry every day. The problem is that food is not distributed properly. Too many people do not have enough money to buy food or own land to grow food themselves.

"Starvation is not a technology problem; it is one of poverty and politics. How will biotech fix that?" asks

Stephen Jones, associate professor and wheat breeder at Washington State University.

Biotechnology proponents claim that genetic engineering will help feed the world by developing more nutritious foods. However, GE crops such as the highly touted "golden rice," which contains higher levels of vitamin A, will not be commercially developed for years. And to date the most widely grown GE crop was developed to withstand sprays of herbicides, not to feed starving people.

Unpredictable Changes

The potential problems from genetic engineering begin with the "shot in the dark" insertion of foreign genes into a plant's DNA. As discussed in Chapter 1, randomly inserted genes may express the desired trait or cause mutations to existing genes of the plant, which produce new toxins or allergens or which reduce the nutritional value of the food.

"When you make a small change in a complex system, the whole system rearranges itself around the change," says Richard Strohman, emeritus professor of molecular and cell biology at the University of California.

Strohman believes that interaction among genes is very complex and should be better understood before genetic engineering can move forward. A lack of understanding about these interactions can lead to unforeseen and possibly negative consequences. "It's difficult to predict the changes that will occur down the road [with genetic engineering]," says Strohman, "they can be negative."

For example, in the mid-1990s, scientists at Pioneer

Hi-Bred seed company introduced a gene from Brazil nuts into soybeans to improve their nutritional content. A University of Nebraska scientist found that the GE soybean would cause allergies in people who are allergic to Brazil nuts. The fearsome prospect was people with the allergy, which can be extremely serious, would not think to avoid eating soybean products.

"No One Has Gotten Sick"

The creation of new allergens is one of the main health risks of GE foods. However, the U.S. government conducts no research on the allergic potential of GE foods, according to a report from the Pew Initiative on Food and Biotechnology. Instead, the government relies on safety data submitted voluntarily by biotechnology companies, an approach that opponents liken to "the fox guarding the hen house."

"There are no tests," says Regal. "The industry claims there are tests, but the data is not there."

"It's misleading to say all genetically engineered products have been tested for safety, it's just not the case," says Mellon. According to the Union of Concerned Scientists, biotechnology companies spend millions of dollars to develop GE crops, but very little is spent to research potential risks.

In June 2000, *Science* magazine reported that an extensive search of scientific journals found just eight articles that studied the safety of GE foods. Of these, only four involved feeding trials. Three of the studies were conducted by Monsanto.

Despite the lack of conclusive scientific study, biotechnology proponents bolster their argument by saying GE foods are subjected to more scientific and regulatory scrutiny than any foods in history and that companies would be foolish to release a GE crop that was not safe to eat. Yet a 2002 report by the Center for Science in the Public Interest (CSPI), an organization focusing on nutrition and food safety, found that the FDA "lacks both the authority and the information to adequately evaluate the safety of GE foods."

Biotechnology companies are not required to submit GE crop safety data to the FDA. They submit such data only voluntarily. The CSPI examined fourteen such submissions from biotech companies, and found that these companies sometimes refused the FDA's requests for more information.

A commonly heard "soundbite" regarding GE foods is "no one has ever gotten sick eating genetically engineered foods." However, it is not actually *known* whether anyone has gotten sick or even died from eating GE foods. As Regal says, "How could you know if someone hasn't gotten sick, if you aren't looking for it?"

For example, several scientists are alarmed about potential health risks of the Cauliflower Mosaic Virus (CaMV) promoter gene, which drives inserted genes to express themselves in GE crops. Dr. Stanley Ewen, a consultant histopathologist at Aberdeen Royal Infirmary in Scotland says the virus is infectious and could increase the risk of stomach and colon cancers. Dr. Mae-Wan Ho, director of the United Kingdom Science in Society, states that the CaMV promoter recombines with other genes to create instability in GE crops and that it has the potential to create new viruses in species to which it is transferred. Ho believes that all GE crops containing CaMV, which includes virtually all of them, should be banned.

Obsolete Basis for Technology

According to Barry Commoner, senior scientist at the Center for the Biology of Natural Systems at Queens College, City University of New York, genetic engineering is based on a scientific theory called the "central dogma," a theory that is forty years old and becoming increasingly obsolete. This theory suggests that there is a one-to-one billiard ball–like relationship between DNA and a protein. Insert a gene and it will produce a protein that expresses the desired trait. However, Commoner cites that recent discoveries, such as that at the Human Genome Project, which found human beings to be made up of far fewer genes than previously predicted, reveal the theory to be flawed. Interactions between genes and proteins are far more complex than previously thought. This complexity explains why genetic engineering produces so many failures, and why only one in 10,000 gene insertions succeeds. As a result, Commoner says, "there are strong reasons to fear the potential consequences of transferring a DNA gene between species."

Chapter 3

UNFORESEEN CONSEQUENCES

"Since neither the U.S. government nor industry appears to be funding any research into the health effects of GE food, the situation is really 'don't look/don't find.'

Perhaps chronic exposure to GE food might be associated with the 70 million incidents each year of 'food poisoning' reported by the government, or with the apparent rises in autism or attention deficit disorder in kids. Or, perhaps not."

—Philip L. Bereano, professor of technology
and public policy, University of Washington,
(editorial, *The Seattle Times*, November 19, 2002).

In October 2000, Jerry Rosman, an Iowa farmer, noticed a problem with his hogs. During breeding, the female sows exhibited all the signs of pregnancy, yet when the time came for them to deliver nothing happened, a phenomenon called "pseudopregnancy." Over the next year, the breeding rates in Rosman's sow herd plummeted 80 percent. Rosman eventually traced the problem back to his feed, which was genetically engineered Bt corn. Laboratory tests revealed that the corn contained high levels of Fusarium mold, indicating possible toxins that could cause disease.

Rosman wasn't the only farmer with the problem. More than twenty farmers in Iowa and surrounding states reported the same breeding problems. Many used the same Bt corn as feed. At least five farmers switched to non-GE corn feed and the problem disappeared.

Rosman's veterinarian said he wouldn't feed the suspect corn to any animal. Scientists at Iowa State University and representatives from the seed company that sold Rosman the corn claimed Bt corn was not the problem. However, the cause was not determined, and Rosman believes some people want to see the problem disappear. "They don't want to admit there is a problem," says Rosman, who blocked sale of the corn, fearing it could cause harm if it entered the food supply. "If this happened here, where else could it happen?"

Rosman has grown GE crops for five years, but he is not so sure he will again. "I've had my eyes opened here," he says.

Jerry Rosman's experience highlights one of the problems with genetic engineering—unforeseen consequences. Scientists know how GE plants function in the laboratory and in field tests but they don't know how they will affect human or animal health and the environment over the long term.

Deadly to Monarch Butterflies?

It is said that a hurricane in the Atlantic Ocean begins when a butterfly in the Sahara Desert flaps its wings. In 1999, a few butterflies eating pollen from GE corn caused a storm of controversy over genetic engineering. Cornell entomologist, John Losey, dusted leaves of the milkweed plant with pollen from Bt corn and fed them to monarch butterfly larvae. Half of the caterpillars fed the leaves containing Bt corn pollen died, while those fed leaves containing pollen from conventional corn survived. In a later study at Iowa State University, this time conducted in actual field conditions, monarch larvae died after eating milkweed leaves containing Bt pollen.

The biotechnology industry responded by funding a series of studies examining the threat of Bt corn to the monarchs. Not surprisingly, the studies found that the corn presented a negligible risk to monarchs. However, in a letter to the U.S. Environmental Protection Agency, Losey and Iowa State University researcher, John Obrycki, said the studies were based on the assumption that monarchs consume only pollen and not other corn tissue, such as anthers. The researchers had found that monarchs do eat anthers, which contain high concentrations of Bt toxins.

StarLink Corn Debacle

In 2000, a hunch that taco shells contained an unapproved GE corn led to a multimillion-dollar food recall. Larry Bohlen, director of health and environment programs at Friends of the Earth, purchased several corn-based products from a Giant supermarket in the Washington, D.C., area and sent them to a laboratory that tests for GE ingredients. Testing revealed that several products contained a Bt corn variety called StarLink that was not approved for human consumption due to concerns that it could cause allergic reactions. The corn entered the food supply because its developer, Aventis Crop-

Science, failed to properly inform farmers of the need to segregate StarLink from other corn and use it as animal feed only.

The discovery led to a massive recall of more than 300 corn products, causing millions of dollars in damages to the agricultural and food industries. The StarLink debacle spawned some thirty lawsuits against Aventis and damaged the reputation of agricultural biotechnology.

Dozens of people reported allergic reactions after eating foods that allegedly contained StarLink corn. Dr. Keith Finger, a Florida optometrist, said he suffered anaphylactic shock, with hives covering ninety percent of his body, after eating a taco shell that contained StarLink.

Potential Health Concerns

Several other incidents and studies have raised concerns about the safety of GE foods:

- **Tryptophan tragedy.** A genetically engineered form of an L-tryptophan food supplement was responsible for the deaths of thirty-seven people and the disabling of several thousand more in 1989. The supplement was genetically engineered by Showa Denko K.K., a Japanese manufacturer. Shortly after the supplement was put on the market, people who took it became ill with Eosinophilia-myalgia syndrome (EMS), a potentially fatal and debilitating disease. The FDA says no definite cause has been established. Showa Denko's laboratory was destroyed, and with it any evidence. But in a September 1991 memo, the FDA's biotechnology coordinator, James Maryanski wrote that the agency could not rule out genetic engineering as the cause.

- **GE potatoes harm rats.** In the late 1990s, Arpad Pusztai, Ph.D., a molecular biologist, conducted a study on genetically engineered potatoes for the Rowett Research Institute in Scotland. The potatoes were genetically engineered to produce lectins, natural insecticides, to protect them against aphids. Pusztai conducted feeding experiments on rats and found that the potatoes damaged the animals' gut, other organs, and immune systems. In 1998, Pusztai expressed his concerns about the transgenic potatoes on a television program, and was promptly suspended and forced to retire from his position. Dr. Pusztai's research was later peer-reviewed and published in *The Lancet*, a leading British medical journal.

- **rBGH risks.** A report conducted by the Canadian Veterinary Medicine Association found that the genetically engineered recombinant bovine growth hormone (rBGH) makes cows more susceptible to infections, diseases, and infertility. As a result of the report, Health Canada, which is Canada's equivalent to the FDA, refused to approve its use. When injected into cows, rBGH stimulates production of a powerful hormone, IGF-1, that is necessary for development but may also stimulate cancers. The major question regarding the safety of rBGH is whether the IGF-1 in milk is absorbed into the human body and leads to elevated levels of the hormone. In addition to Canada, the European Union has banned the use of rBGH due to health risks.

- **GE gene transfers to human gut.** In 2002, British scientists found that genetically engineered material in foods can transfer to human gut bacteria. The biotechnology industry has insisted that such "horizontal gene transfers" to human beings are not possible. Horizontal gene transfers could create new viruses and bacteria that cause disease. In particular, concerns have been raised about antibiotic-resistant marker genes that are inserted into GE crops. Scientists fear that marker genes could transfer antibiotic resistance to humans, animals, and pathogens, rendering antibiotic medicines ineffective.

- **Reduced nutrition in GE soybeans.** A study conducted by the Center for Ethics and Toxics and published in the *Journal of Medicinal Food* found that the levels of phytoestrogens (naturally occurring plant compounds with known health benefits) in GE soybeans were 12 to 14 percent less than those in conventional soybeans.

The Institute for Science in Society says the increased consumption of GE foods could be a cause for the two- to tenfold increase in food-related illnesses in the United States between 1994 and 1999. The majority of these illnesses and food-related deaths were caused by unknown agents.

Environmental Concerns

Genetic engineering has given new meaning to the word "contamination" as engineered genes from transgenic plants proliferate in the environment and "pollute" organic and conventional crops and other plant life.

Unlike chemical pollutants that can be contained or mitigated, genetic pollutants multiply in the environment and cannot be recalled or contained.

Contamination occurs when pollen from GE crops such as corn and canola is carried by wind or insects and cross-pollinates with similar crops or weeds. In these cases, a GE trait, such as herbicide resistance, could pass to related plants and create "superweeds." Canola farmers in Canada have reported that such herbicide-resistant weeds are becoming a problem. In Manitoba, three GE canola varieties cross-pollinated with a weed, making it triple herbicide-resistant.

A study by Allison Snow, professor of evolution, ecology, and organismal biology at Ohio State University, found that the Bt gene has the potential to migrate to weeds and strengthen them. Snow studied GE sunflowers and found they could crossbreed with nearby weedy relatives. "Weeds are already hardy plants, and the addition of transgenes could make them just tougher," says Snow.

In a 2001 paper published in *Nature* magazine, at the University of California at Berkeley, researchers Ignacio Chapela and David Quist described how genes from GE corn contaminated native corn varieties in Oaxaca, Mexico. The finding was particularly disturbing because contamination was found thousands of miles from plantings of GE corn, and because it threatened the center of biological diversity for corn. The discovery angered proponents of biotechnology who claimed the study was flawed and attempted to discredit Chapela and Quist. However, subsequent research by the Mexican government and the Mexican National Institute of Ecology confirmed the presence of genetically engineered DNA in the corn varieties.

Gene flow from GE canola and corn to organic crops has resulted in economic losses for organic farmers who cannot sell the contaminated crops. Organic canola is no longer grown in Canada due to gene flow from GE canola, resulting in an estimated loss of several hundred thousand dollars per year to farmers.

An editorial in *Nature Biotechnology*, a leading industry journal, warned biotechnology companies, "Gene flow from crops to related plants thus remains a concern for regulators, and one that companies need to address. . . . It is time that industry took decisive steps to address gene flow from their products. Environmental concerns surrounding GM crops are not going to go away."

Killer GE Bacterium

One major environmental concern was raised in the early 1990s with a potentially devastating GE bacterium. At that time, German scientists, aiming to eliminate the need to burn fields and thereby cause pollution, engineered a soil bacterium called *Klebsiella planticola*, to break down crop debris into alcohol. The U.S. Environmental Protection Agency approved the GE bacterium for field-testing. However, research by Elaine Ingham, a soil microbiologist at Oregon State University, and a graduate student found that the GE bacterium killed all living wheat plants to which it was added. Based on the findings, Ingham believes that if the fast-spreading bacterium was released into the environment, it could enter root systems and kill plant life—everywhere. Ingham states, "This could have been the single most devastating impact on human beings since we would likely have lost corn, wheat, barley, vegetable crops, trees, bushes, etc, conceivably all terrestrial plants." The EPA conducted its own research on the bacterium, and never approved it for field testing.

No Insurance, Research Obstacles

The health and environmental risks of transgenic foods are potentially so great that insurance companies refuse to offer full coverage to biotechnology companies. Switzerland-based reinsurance company Rueck, the world's second largest reinsurance company, concluded in a 1998 study that there was no way to evaluate the health and environmental risks of genetic engineering and thus offer appropriate coverage.

Research highlighting the risks of genetically engineered crops to human health and the environment faces obstacles because such studies go against the grain in a political and corporate climate that favors and promotes biotechnology. For example, Pioneer Hi-Bred International and Dow AgroSciences eliminated funding for Allison Snow's research on gene transfer to weeds shortly after she published her findings. When such research does get published, biotech proponents and scientists, perceiving a threat to their scientific paradigm, viciously attack both the study and the researchers. Scientists, such as Arpad Pusztai, have been discredited, and even lost their jobs. Ignacio Chapela was refused tenure by the University of California after he discovered GE contamination in Mexico's native corn varieties.

Chapter 4

BIOTECH—THE NEXT GENERATION: "PHARMA," "GOLDEN RICE," AND GE ANIMALS

*"Just one mistake by a biotech company,
and we'll be eating other people's prescription
drugs in our corn flakes."*

—Larry Bohlen, director of health and environment programs,
Friends of the Earth

On a November day in 2002, five members of the environmental group Greenpeace climbed a grain elevator in Aurora, Nebraska, and unfurled a 30- by 40-foot banner that featured a syringe injected into an ear of corn with the message, "This is your food on drugs. Ban genetically engineered drug crops." The grain elevator stored a controversial harvest— a small amount of a corn genetically engineered to produce a pharmaceutical substance. The corn had accidentally mixed with 500,000 bushels of soybeans, and the U.S. Department of Agriculture (USDA) ordered the elevator quarantined to prevent the experimental corn from entering the food supply. The corn's developer, ProdiGene, based in College Station, Texas, was forced to destroy the soybeans and paid $3 million in fines and penalties to the USDA for mishandling the corn.

The controversy signaled the next generation of genetically engineered crops, "pharma" or "plant-made pharmaceuticals." Biotechnology companies are genetically engineering plants, such as corn and tobacco, to produce pharmaceutical and industrial substances. Prodi-Gene is developing several pharma-corn varieties to produce drugs and an industrial enzyme. In 2002 the company contracted a group of farmers to grow the crops on a few hundred acres in the Midwestern United States. Another company, Epicyte Pharmaceutical Inc., based in San Diego, is genetically engineering corn to develop a drug that prevents the transmission of the herpes virus. Other pharma crops under development include one that will produce antibodies for therapeutic blood products and oral vaccines for human and animal diseases. A study by the National Corn Growers Association found that some 400 plant-based drugs are being developed worldwide.

Fears of Drugs Entering the Food Supply

Biotech companies use corn to develop pharma products because it costs less to grow and can produce larger quantities than other plants. However, Allison Snow, a biologist at Ohio State University and an expert on cross-pollination, says corn is the worst plant species to use because it disperses pollen far and wide. Environmental and food industry groups fear that pharma crops will contaminate food crops and enter the food supply where they could cause toxic or allergic reactions in human beings. "We need to think really hard about putting drugs in corn, which is highly out-crossing, (cross-pollinating) " says Margaret Mellon of the Union of Concerned Scientists. "Neighboring farmers may harvest pharma crops even though they planted conventional seed."

According to the Genetically Engineered Food Alert, more than 300 open-air field trials of pharma crops have been conducted in unidentified locations across the United States

The National Academy of Sciences warned that "it is possible that crops transformed to produce pharmaceutical or other industrial compounds might mate with plantations grown for human consumption, with the unanticipated result of novel chemicals in the human food supply."

ProdiGene claims to have an "identity containment" system in place to isolate pharma crops and prevent cross-pollination. The system includes isolating the crops far from food crops, inspecting fields, and using dedicated equipment for planting, harvesting, and storage. However, Fred Kirschenmann, director of the Leopold Center for Sustainable Agriculture at Iowa State University, doubts that pollen can be contained. "Organisms in nature have developed ingenious means of dispersing themselves and to assume that one can maintain an enclave to prevent that is a stretch," says Kirschenmann. "What is the scientific basis for claiming that this crop can be contained?"

Indeed, ProdiGene's mishap in Nebraska, and another in Iowa, when a test plot of pharma corn contaminated a nearby field, revealed gaping holes in the containment strategy.

ProdiGene's near disasters alarmed the powerful

food industry whose representatives demanded zero tolerance of food contamination by pharma crops. Industry representatives also lobbied the government to prohibit the use of food crops to produce pharma products. In 2003, the USDA responded by introducing stricter rules, including a one-mile separation between pharma and non-GE crops, but food and environmental groups criticized the rules as inadequate.

Doubts remain. Have other pharma crops, which have been grown on hundreds of acres, slipped past USDA inspectors and entered the food supply? No one knows. The answer, to quote a famous line by Bob Dylan, "is blowin' in the wind."

Biotech Pipeline

Scientists worldwide are developing hundreds of other transgenic crops in the hopes that they will benefit humanity. Whether they will or not remains to be seen. The most famous is "golden rice," which is genetically engineered to produce beta-carotene and increase vitamin A levels. Each year vitamin A deficiencies are said to cause death and blindness to thousands of children in developing countries. Development of golden rice sparked heated debate between proponents and opponents of GE foods. Jeremy Rifkin, founder and president of the Foundation on Economic Trends and noted biotech critic, calls golden rice "pure public relations" from the biotech industry. Gordon Conway, president of the Rockefeller Foundation, which helped fund golden rice research, argues that it would provide 15 to 20 percent of the daily requirement for vitamin A, which would be helpful. Golden rice is currently undergoing safety and nutrition tests in the Philippines and is expected to be available by 2005.

Below are a few examples of other GE crops that are being developed:

- **Hypoallergenic wheat.** Scientists at the University of California at Berkeley are genetically engineering wheat to reduce its allergenic properties.

- **Hypoallergenic rice.** Biotech company Syngenta has genetically engineered rice to remove a protein that triggers allergic reactions. The rice is designed to help kidney dialysis patients in Asia who cannot tolerate the high protein content of local rice.

- **Cancer-fighting tomato.** Scientists at Purdue University and the USDA genetically engineered tomatoes to ripen later, giving them longer shelf life. The tomatoes also contain higher levels of lycopene, a substance that has been associated with reducing the risk of prostate cancer in men.

- **Disease-resistant sweet potato.** African scientists genetically engineered a sweet potato to resist a virus that consumes more than three-fourths of the harvest in Kenya. However, the GE sweet potato failed to resist the virus in field tests.

- **Salt-water crops.** Chinese scientists say they have isolated the gene that allows certain vegetation to thrive in salt water. They hope the discovery will enable them to develop crops that grow in salt-water areas.

- **Higher protein potato.** Scientists in India have added a gene to potatoes, which, they say, makes the plant produce more protein and essential amino acids.

- **Edible vaccine.** Researchers at The Boyce Thompson Institute for plant research at Cornell University are modifying bananas to produce a hepatitis B vaccine.

Other GE crops in the "pipeline" include Roundup Ready versions of wheat, alfalfa, lettuce, tomato, and golf-course turf grass, Bt apples, disease-resistant bananas, and herbicide-resistant rice and strawberries. Many of these GE crops are five to 10 years away from entering the market, and face significant hurdles including the substantial costs of commercialization, regulatory requirements, and potential market rejection.

The number of new GE crops entering the market has slowed in recent years because of increasing consumer concerns over their safety, as well as their rejection in Europe and other nations. In 1998, the FDA approved thirteen new GE crops, but by 2002 that number dropped to two.

Margaret Mellon questions the need to create more nutritious foods through genetic engineering. "We have a cornucopia of nutritious foods already available," she says. "Conventional breeding can enhance nutrition levels." The need, she says, is not more good foods, but educating consumers about the benefits of eating a good diet.

GE Animals

Scientists in Italy have manipulated swine sperm to create pigs that have human genes in their hearts, livers, and kidneys. The aim is to produce a breed of pigs with organs that could be removed for transplants into human beings. A Canadian company has inserted spider genes into female goats so they express spider silk proteins in their milk, which would be used to create strong fiber. Livestock breeders in the United States have produced hundreds of cloned animals, including milk cows and pigs. In 1997 Scottish scientists cloned the first animal, a sheep named Dolly, then later crossed the embryos of a goat and a sheep to create a "geep," an animal with the head of a goat and body of a sheep.

Massachusetts-based Aqua Bounty Farms has genetically engineered salmon to grow twice as fast as conventional salmon. Environmentalists say the transgenic salmon could escape from fish farm pens and interbreed with wild salmon, threatening the species. The FDA is reviewing an application by Aqua Bounty farms to market the salmon. Meanwhile, 200 chefs, grocers, and seafood distributors have pledged not to purchase the transgenic salmon, and Washington State has banned GE fish from its waters.

In 2002, the National Academy of Sciences released a report stating that genetic manipulation of animals poses serious risks to the environment and to human health. The report said that the escape of GE animals into to the wild could alter species or even wipe them out. In addition, the report said that, unless it is managed carefully, the introduction of GE meat, milk, or eggs could harm human health.

Chapter 5

FIGHTING FOR
THE RIGHT TO KNOW

*"You have a right to know what you eat, especially when
it's better... After several months of debate, Europe
has just adopted a new law for the labeling of food
that comes from genetically engineered plants....
We believe that products that come from biotechnology
are better and that they should be labeled."*

—Text from Monsanto advertisement that appeared
in French magazines in 1998.

Mel Bankoff firmly believes foods containing genetically engineered ingredients should be labeled.
"Consumers having the right to know what is in their
food cuts through the public relations promotion of the
biotech companies," says Bankoff, president of Emerald
Valley Kitchen, an organic food company in Eugene, Oregon. Bankoff's passion led him to spearhead a 2002 state-
wide ballot initiative known as Measure 27 to label GE
foods in the state of Oregon.

FDA Policy: No Labeling

The Oregon group resorted to a ballot measure because
the FDA refuses to require specific labeling of foods with

GE ingredients, which, despite the risks, are found in about 70 percent of processed foods. The FDA's policy, which was established in 1992, states that foods developed by genetic engineering are "substantially equivalent" to those produced by traditional plant breeding. Labeling would be required only if a GE ingredient alters the nutritional content, health, or safety of the food product. As a result, the agency doesn't require labeling, and safety testing is voluntary for the companies that produce them.

Biotech companies and the food industry support the FDA's policy and argue that mandatory labeling would be costly and act as a "skull and crossbones" to scare off consumers.

Bankoff sees it differently. "Biotech companies have done a stealth attack on the market without full disclosure," he says. "If their product is as great as they claim, why not allow people to know what it is, and put in on the front panel?"

The FDA, says Bankoff, "has put corporate profitability over health and environmental concerns."

FDA Scientists Voiced Concerns

The FDA's policy on GE foods was developed during the presidential administrations of Ronald Reagan and George Bush, who emphasized the need to "get the government off the backs of businesses." The government's position reflects that stance by essentially letting biotechnology companies regulate themselves.

However, internal FDA documents reveal that the agency's own scientists have expressed strong doubts about FDA policy on GE foods, and have simultaneously raised questions about the foods' safety.

The FDA's policy states, "The agency is not aware of any information showing that foods derived by these new (genetic engineering) methods differ from other foods in any meaningful or uniform way, or that, as a class, foods developed by the new technologies present any different or greater safety concern than foods developed by traditional plant breeding."

Yet in a February 1992 memo, Louis J. Pribyl, Ph.D., a scientist in the FDA's Microbiology Group, critiqued a draft of the policy by writing, "There is a profound difference between the types of unexpected effects from traditional breeding and genetic engineering which is just glanced over in this document." Dr. Pribyl added that several aspects of gene insertion "may be more hazardous than traditional plant crossbreeding."

Linda Kahl, Ph.D., an FDA compliance officer, emphasized the lack of required scientific data to establish the safety of GE foods. "Are we asking the scientific experts to generate the basis for this policy statement in the absence of any data?" she wrote, "There is no data that could quantify risk."

E. J. Matthews, Ph.D., of the FDA's Toxicology group warned in an October 1991 memo, "Genetically modified plants could also contain unexpected high concentrations of plant toxicants."

Consumers Want Labeling

Despite the FDA's refusal to label GE foods, surveys consistently show that a majority of American consumers favor labeling. A 2002 survey conducted by the Food Policy Institute at Rutgers University found that 90 percent of consumers say that GE foods should be labeled. A 2003 poll by ABCNEWS.com showed that 92 percent of respondents think GE foods should be labeled. A 2001 survey by the Pew Initiative on Food and Biotechnology found that 75 percent of Americans said it was important for them to know whether a food contained GE ingredients and 46 percent said it was very important for them to know.

Even the FDA's own consumer focus groups on GE foods found that, "Virtually all participants said that bio-engineered foods should be labeled as such." In addition, most focus group participants expressed outrage when they were informed of how pervasive GE foods are. Many complained that GE foods had been "snuck in" to the food supply without their knowledge and were disturbed by the lack of public information about a major change in their foods.

Proposed Legislation

Legislation to label GE foods has been introduced at the national and state levels. In 1999, Representative Dennis Kucinich (D-Ohio) introduced The Genetically Engineered Food Right to Know Act (HR 3377). The bill attracted fifty-seven cosponsors but never came up for a vote in the House. Senator Barbara Boxer (D-California) introduced similar legislation in the Senate.

Kucinich reintroduced the bill in 2003 along with five other bills related to GE foods. The bills aim to ensure that consumers are protected, increase food safety, protect farmers' rights, make biotech companies liable for their products, and help developing nations resolve hunger concerns. "This issue is gaining a higher profile," says Kucinich. "People have a right to know so they can make appropriate choices for their own health."

Though Congress has yet to act on the labeling legislation, Kucinich is dedicated to getting it passed. "We're going to put the bill out and continue our efforts to get it to the American people," he says.

Groups that back labeling of GE foods include the Consumer Federation of America, the American Association of Retired Persons (AARP), the Sierra Club, the National Farmers Organization, the Center for Food Safety, the Organic Trade Organization, and the American Corn Growers Association.

Hank Jenkins-Smith, professor of political science at the University of New Mexico, says the labeling issue is "potentially explosive." "People want the choice. They don't mind taking risks, but they want to be the ones who choose," he says. Jenkins-Smith and researchers at Texas A&M conducted a two-year study on consumer attitudes toward GE foods.

Goes against Global Trend

While the United States and Canada refuse to require mandatory labeling of GE foods, more than forty nations either require labeling or are developing labeling laws. These nations include the fifteen European Union member states: Russia, the Czech Republic, Slovakia, Slovenia, Switzerland, China, Japan, South Korea, Thailand, Taiwan, South Africa, Israel, Saudi Arabia, Indonesia, and Brazil.

It is ironic that governments known to be repressive,

such as China and Russia, give their consumers the right to know whether foods contain GE ingredients, whereas the United States, which claims to be the champion of human rights, does not.

Labeling laws require that foods containing GE ingredients above a certain percentage be labeled as genetically engineered. The "tolerances" vary from nation to nation. There is no agreed-upon "safe" tolerance. A strict tolerance is considered to be 0.1%. This minute percentage is based upon what regulators believe is the acceptable amount of contamination allowed in foods. Food products in the European Union that contain GE ingredients above 0.9 percent must be labeled while foods in Japan that contain more than 5 percent GE ingredients must carry labels.

"Gag Manufacturers" of Organic, Non-GE Products

Many natural and organic product companies want to inform consumers that their products don't contain GE ingredients. They accomplish this by labeling their products "GE-Free," "contains no genetically modified organisms" (GMOs), or "non-GMO."

Organic food manufacturers say their consumers want to know if the product contains GE ingredients. "We are absolutely convinced there is a market segment that wants this information," says Steven Demos, president, White Wave, Inc., a leading manufacturer of organic soymilk.

Surveys confirm Demos's belief. The Center for Science in the Public Interest found that 31 percent of consumers surveyed would prefer food labels stating "does not contain genetically engineered ingredients" to the absence of labels.

In 2001, the FDA introduced a draft guidance document to help companies label their products as non-GMO. However, the document restricts wording that can be used on labels. Instead of commonly used acronyms such as "non-GMO" or "non-GE," companies may be required to use phrases like "We do not use ingredients that were produced using biotechnology" or "This oil is made from soybeans that weren't genetically engineered."

Organic product manufacturers are unhappy with the FDA's recommendations. Michael Potter, president of Eden Foods and Arran Stephens, president of Nature's Path Foods, both say the burden of labeling—with its added costs of ensuring that no GE ingredients contaminate their products—is wrongly placed on organic manufacturers instead of biotechnology companies. "Not only is the FDA failing to mandate labeling of genetically engineered foods, but now they want to gag manufacturers of products that don't contain GMOs (genetically modified organisms)," says Potter.

Stephens says that the FDA's proposals on labeling non-GE foods are incomprehensible. "We go to great lengths to keep GMOs out of our products and should have the democratic right to label our products as such," says Stephens. "Mandatory labeling of GE foods is needed."

Mel Bankoff sees genetic engineering as an assault against the organic industry. "With the proliferation of genetically engineered crops, organic won't be able to survive. There's no way to stop contamination once these genes get into the pollen," he says.

Measure 27: The Battle of Oregon

Frustrated by the lack of government action, Bankoff and the Oregon Concerned Citizens for Safe Foods decided to take the issue directly to the voters of Oregon. The group collected more than 97,000 petition signatures, which was 31,000 more than the 66,000 needed to get the initiative on the ballot for the state's election.

Bankoff helped fund the initiative with a contribution of $50,000 that helped pay for radio and television ads. He was a leading spokesman for the pro-labeling group, wrote a newspaper editorial arguing for Measure 27, and persuaded former Beatle, Sir Paul McCartney, to record a radio ad supporting labeling. "Let it be labeled," said McCartney.

Measure 27 was a classic "David and Goliath" fight with consumers, environmental groups, and organic food manufacturers supporting the initiative on one side and agricultural and food industry groups opposing it on the other. Supporters hoped that passage of Measure 27 would lead other states, such as California, to adopt labeling, starting a trend that would sweep across the nation. The opposition, known as the Coalition Against the Costly Label Law included farm and food industry groups who argued that labeling would cost the average consumer an extra $550 per year for food. However, a study by William K. Jaeger, an agricultural economist at Oregon State University, estimated that labeling would cost between $0.23 and $10 per person per year.

Thanks to deep pockets, the opposition communicated their message more effectively. Major food manufacturers and biotechnology companies, including General

Mills, Kellogg Company, Monsanto and DuPont, spent more than $5 million in advertising to persuade Oregonians to vote against Measure 27. The total was the most ever spent to defeat a ballot initiative in Oregon and amounted to more than the combined campaign money spent by Oregon's two gubernatorial candidates. Such heavy spending indicated the corporations' fear of GE food labeling. Significantly, only about $5,500 of the opposition's millions came from Oregon companies; the rest was from multinational corporations. On the other hand, Measure 27 supporters raised about $194,000 or less than 5 percent as much as the opposition.

Big money carried the day: Measure 27 was defeated with 73 percent voting against and 27 percent voting in favor. Despite the defeat, Bankoff says the fight for labeling will continue. "This is not the end, only the beginning of the debate in both Oregon and nationwide."

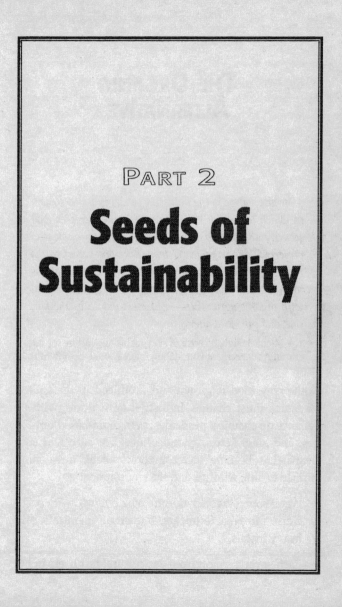

PART 2

Seeds of
Sustainability

Chapter 6

THE ORGANIC ALTERNATIVE

"The alternative to the industrial model is a food system in which food trade raises incomes, and increases food security at both ends; one in which the environment is preserved; one in which farmers have fair access to the means of food production and consumers have fair access to food at fair prices. These principles are best associated with organic agriculture—which set out to be the fair, safe, and sane food alternative."

—Michael Sligh, director of sustainable agriculture for the Rural Advancement Foundation International–USA (RAFI)

The way food is grown and produced in the United States must change. Industrial agriculture, with its reliance on chemical pesticides, petroleum-based fertilizers, and single crop "monocultures" of corn and soybeans, has become increasingly obsolete, threatening human health, wildlife, and the environment:

- Water sources worldwide are now polluted with pesticides, nitrogen fertilizers, industrial chemicals, and heavy metals.

- Each spring, runoff from agricultural fertilizers in the

Midwest creates a "dead zone" in the Gulf of Mexico near the Mississippi Delta where fish die because of too little oxygen. The dead zone covers more than 7,000 square miles—an area the size of New Jersey.

- More than 1 million children between the ages of one and five ingest at least fifteen pesticides every day from fruits and vegetables. More than 600,000 of these children eat a dose of insecticides that the U.S. government considers unsafe.

- Nearly one-third of the world's arable land has been lost to erosion, and the United States has lost three-fourths of all agricultural diversity.

- Pesticide use on major field crops, fruits, and vegetables nearly tripled, rising from 215 million pounds in 1964 to 588 million pounds in 1997, while the number of insects known to be resistant to pesticides has more than tripled, increasing from 137 in 1962 to more than 500 by the late 1980s.

In a study published in *Science*, University of Minnesota ecologist David Tilman and colleagues concluded that continued expansion of industrial farming for the next few decades "has the potential to have massive, irreversible environmental impacts" and expose humans to markedly higher levels of pesticides.

Proponents of biotechnology claim that genetically engineered crops will reduce the need for agricultural pesticides. The claim lacks credibility because the biotechnology companies that produce GE crops also produced the chemicals that created the current problems. If the companies' claims about the safety of agricultural chemicals were false, how can anyone believe their claims that GE foods will also be safe?

There is an alternative and that is organic agriculture.

Ancient and Modern

Over the last fifty years, organic agriculture emerged as a sustainable solution to the hazards of industrial agriculture. According to the United States National Organic Standards Board, organic agriculture "is an ecological production management system that promotes and enhances biodiversity, biological cycles and soil biological activity. It is based on minimal use of off-farm inputs and on management practices that restore, maintain and enhance ecological harmony. The primary goal of organic agriculture is to optimize the health and productivity of interdependent communities of soil life, plants, animals and people."

Organic agriculture has its roots in farming practices used for centuries by indigenous peoples throughout the world. The modern organic agriculture movement was started in the 1940s by Paul Keene, founder of Walnut Acres farm, and J. I. Rodale, publisher of *Organic Gardening and Farming*, the first magazine to focus on organic farming. Publication of Rachel Carson's book, *Silent Spring*, in 1962 which chronicled the environmental damage of industrial agriculture, spurred interest in organic methods. Farmers and researchers began to recognize organic agriculture's commonsense approach with its emphasis on improving the health of the soil, plants, animals, and human beings, without the use of hazardous chemicals. The organic movement grew steadily during the later part of the twentieth century, as organic certification and farming organizations, such as Maine Organic Farmers and Gardeners Association and California Certified Organic Farmers, were formed and sales of organic foods increased.

Intelligent System

Organic agriculture is not a primitive, "back to the land" fad, but a viable, intelligent, and effective way to produce foods. Organic practitioners employ beneficial advances, such as new crop varieties and machinery, while discarding methods, such as the use of chemical pesticides, that cause negative effects to human health and the environment.

Such a system requires intelligent planning and methods. While industrial farmers use synthetic fertilizers, organic farmers employ crop rotations, cover crops, and compost to enhance soil fertility. To manage weeds without using toxic herbicides, organic farmers use beneficial allelopathic plants that limit weed growth, cultivation, mulching with straw or wood chips, and propane flame burning. The farmer's aim is to increase the beneficial insects that keep pests in check. Instead of pesticides, organic farmers use biological, cultural, and physical methods to limit pests, simultaneously aiming to increase the beneficial insects that keep pests in check. Seed varieties are bred to resist insects and disease.

In his book, *The Botany of Desire*, Michael Pollan contrasted the approaches of two Idaho potato farmers, one conventional, the other organic. The conventional farmer grew Russet Burbank potatoes, which are favored by processors of French fries, but susceptible to the leafroll virus that causes a brown spotting. To kill the virus, the farmer must spray his fields with a highly toxic pesticide called Monitor. Meanwhile, the organic farmer completely avoids the problem by growing potato varieties that don't attract the virus. Such preventative measures are key to organic farming.

Organic Gets Its Seal of Approval

Organic foods must be certified, which means they must have been grown and produced according to strict standards developed by organic certification organizations. In 2002, these standards were unified under the USDA's National Organic Program. The goal of the national program is to standardize production of organic foods, and give a consistent meaning to the term "organic."

Establishing the National Organic Program was a long and challenging process. In the 1980s, organic industry leaders lobbied the U.S. government to establish national standards. Unlike most industries that want to avoid regulations, the organic industry *asked* the government for them. Prior to the National Organic Program, organic food was certified through a patchwork of independent organizations and state agencies, each with its own standards for producing organic products. As a result, the term "organic" had no consistent meaning from state to state, or from certifier to certifier. The term was used loosely and sometimes falsely to the frustration of organic farmers and processors. In 1990, Congress passed the Organic Foods Production Act, which mandated rules for the production, handling, and marketing of organic foods.

In 1997, the USDA issued proposed rules allowing the use of irradiation, sewer sludge, and genetic engineering in organic foods. Outraged consumers flooded the USDA with 275,000 letters protesting the proposals, which forced the agency to prohibit these controversial suggestions being accepted for organic farming.

The National Organic Program also prohibits the use of antibiotics and growth hormones, as well as chemical insecticides, herbicides, fungicides, and fertilizers, in organic dairy, meat, and poultry. Farmers must plant organic seed. Organic crops must be rotated to maintain soil health. Animals raised to produce organic dairy, meat, and poultry must be fed organic feed.

The National Organic Program was finally implemented on October 21, 2002, and foods certified organic were permitted to display the green and white "USDA Organic" seal. The achievement represented a significant milestone for the organic industry and promised to fuel even greater demand for organic foods.

Consumers Prefer Organic

Today's health-conscious American consumers see organic foods as a healthier alternative to conventional and genetically engineered foods. A 2002 study by National Marketing Institute found that 39 percent of the United States' population, over 40 million households, uses organic products. A 2002 study by the Food Marketing Institute (FMI) and *Prevention* magazine found that more than 60 percent of American shoppers believe that organic foods are better for their health. In contrast only 37 percent believe genetically engineered foods are acceptable, and 65 percent said that scientists don't know enough yet to control the effects of genetic engineering.

The Question of Cost

Organic foods can cost as much as 25 percent more than conventional foods, depending on the season and availability of a product. There are several reasons for this. Farmers must meet strict standards for certification, and organic production requires more labor. In addition, organic crops are grown on a smaller scale, which means farmers may pay more per acre to produce them. Unlike many conventional farmers, organic farmers do not receive government subsidies to support their efforts. Finally, when the costs needed to address and repair the damaging side effects of industrial agriculture—to clean up polluted waters, replace eroded soils, and provide health care for farmers and workers—are factored into the price of food, organic foods would cost the same or even less than conventional foods.

Organic farming leaders aim to lower the cost of organic foods. "This movement did not start out to establish expensive niche-market foods for rich people, but to model an alternative system for all of agriculture," says Michael Sligh. "We must make this accessible for all people."

Fastest-Growing Segment

What started as a sprout more than sixty years ago has blossomed into a multibillion-dollar industry. Organic is the fastest-growing segment of the United States food industry with demand increasing by 20 percent each year since 1990. Sales of organic products in the United States are projected to grow from $9.35 billion in 2001 to $20 billion by 2005. Despite the growth, organic food accounts for just 1 percent of total food production in the United States.

According to the USDA's Economic Research Service, between 1997 and 2001 certified organic farm acreage grew from 1.35 million to 2.23 million acres, an addition of 1 million acres, a more than 140 percent increase. The number of farmers certified organic is now over 5,000.

Worldwide organic acreage now tops 54 million. Australia leads the world with 26 million acres, followed by Argentina with 8 million, Italy with 3 million, and then the United States with 2.23 million. However, the United States ranks thirty-sixth among all nations in percentage of agricultural land for organic use with just 0.2 percent. Germany aims to convert 20 percent of its arable land to organic by 2010. Belgium and the Netherlands plan to convert 10 percent to organic by the same year. The United States has no such goals. In fact, the USDA devotes *less than one-tenth of 1 percent* of its research budget to organic projects.

Problems with "Big Organic"

The booming demand for organic food has attracted major food companies. General Mills, Kellogg Company, HJ Heinz, Proctor & Gamble, and Kraft Foods have either launched organic brands or purchased organic food companies. HJ Heinz sells an organic version of its venerable ketchup. Fast-food giant McDonald's introduced organic milk into its restaurants in Great Britain.

Organic industry leaders express mixed feelings about

the entry of large corporations. Some say the big names will increase public acceptance of organic foods and expand the market even more; however, others fear the companies may attempt to weaken the strict standards that have been the hallmark of organic production.

In fact, one corporation attempted to change the organic rules to suit its own ends. In February 2003, Fieldale Farms Corp., a poultry producer based in Baldwin, Georgia, lobbied Congress for an exemption to the rule requiring that organic feed be given to animals raised to produce organic meat and dairy products. In a classic example of backroom political maneuvering, Georgia Congressman Nathan Deal slipped a provision into a 3,000-page congressional spending bill that would override the requirement for organic feed if a government study found that organic feed costs twice as much as non-organic. With the one-sentence "rider," Congressman Deal, backed by Congress, attempted to gut twelve years of work to develop the organic standards. The *St. Petersburg Times* described Deal's action as "a sleazy political favor."

Fortunately, the organic industry backed by Senator Patrick Leahy (D-VT) led a successful effort to repeal Deal's rider.

Unfortunately, this may be the first of other corporate or government attempts to weaken the organic standards and the integrity of organic foods. Such attacks threaten an industry that has proven to be socially and environmentally responsible, economically vital, and beneficial to consumers.

Chapter 7

A HEALTHY ARGUMENT FOR ORGANIC

"I didn't switch to organic farming for the money
or a utopian dream. I did it for myself and
my family in order to stay in agriculture."

—Blaine Schmaltz, North Dakota organic wheat farmer

Some farmers switch to growing organic crops to be better stewards of the land. Others make the transition to earn the premium prices paid for organic. For Blaine Schmaltz the decision to become an organic farmer was a life-saving necessity.

"You Won't Live 10 Years"

Schmaltz, a wheat farmer from Rugby, North Dakota, had always been sensitive to agricultural chemicals. As a boy, he sometimes got sick and vomited when exposed to them. Despite the sensitivity he continued using the chemicals as he grew older. One day in September 1993, it became too much. Schmaltz was spraying an herbicide on his field. At one point he looked inside the sprayer tank to check the level. Then he passed out. Neighbors found him lying in a ditch. They revived him, and Schmaltz made his way home, but he developed asthma, suffered muscle aches and pains, and couldn't sleep. Later that winter he was hospitalized.

At first, doctors couldn't target a specific disease, then one finally diagnosed Schmaltz as having "occupational asthma." "The doctor told me to leave agriculture," he says. "He said, 'if you don't you probably won't live ten years.'"

"Did This in Respect to My Health"

Schmaltz faced a crisis. "It was scary because I had four young children, had given up my job, and made an investment in the farm," he says.

During that same winter while recovering from his illness, Schmaltz began reading about organic farming. "I thought if I could get rid of the hazardous things that bothered me, I could stay with the occupation I loved dearly," he says.

The next spring Schmaltz began the transition to organic farming, and over time, discovered it was the right choice. His symptoms disappeared. "It worked," he says. "I substituted more natural alternatives for the chemicals and they didn't bother me."

Today, Schmaltz operates a successful organic farm growing wheat, edible beans, and other grains. "I did this in respect to my health," says Schmaltz. "It's been hard work but it has been rewarding and meaningful."

Pesticide Health Hazards

Blaine Schmaltz's life-threatening experience with agricultural chemicals is one of thousands reported each year. The Environmental Protection Agency estimates there are 10,000 to 20,000 physician-diagnosed pesticide illnesses and injuries per year in farm work. A 2001 U.S. government study found that "Exposure to pesticides can cause a range of ill effects in humans, from relatively mild effects such as headaches, fatigue, and nausea, to more serious effects such as cancer and neurological disorders."

Pesticide residues are everywhere—in our air, soil, water, food, and our bodies. A study by researchers at the University of Missouri-Columbia found that men living in agricultural areas had sperm counts as much as 40 percent lower than men living in major cities, such as New York and Los Angeles. Runoff from farm chemicals is the suspected cause. A study by the Pesticide Action Network found that United States' consumers could experience up to seventy daily exposures to residues from persistent organic pollutants (POPs) through their diets. Exposure to POPs, which are among the most dangerous compounds ever produced, has been linked to breast and other types of cancer, immune system suppression, nervous system disorders, reproductive damage, and disruption of hormonal systems.

Less Exposure to Pesticides

The obvious way to prevent health problems caused by pesticides, as Blaine Schmaltz discovered, is to switch to organic agriculture. Research confirms this view. An extensive study conducted by the Organic Materials Review Institute and Consumers Union, publisher of *Consumer Reports* magazine, confirmed that organic foods contain significantly fewer pesticides than conventionally produced foods. Researchers analyzed test data in more than 94,000 organic and nonorganic food samples of about twenty different crops tested over nearly a decade. Results showed that 73 percent of conventionally grown produce had at least one pesticide residue, while only 23 percent of organically grown samples contained residues. In California, pesticide residues were found in nearly a third of conventionally grown foods, compared to just 6.5 percent of organic samples. Considering the widespread nature of pesticides, these numbers are very low. "We can now say with confidence that organic farming systems help reduce exposure to pesticides in the human diet," says Charles Benbrook, an agricultural economist and coauthor of the study.

A study conducted by researchers at the University of Washington's School of Public Health and Community Medicine, found that preschool children eating a diet of organic foods had six to nine times lower pesticide levels in their bodies than children eating conventional foods. The authors concluded, "Consumption of organic produce appears to provide a relatively simple means for parents to reduce their children's exposure to organophosphorus pesticides."

Increased Nutrition

Research is also finding that organic foods offer health benefits beyond exposure to pesticides. Studies comparing the nutritional value of organic and conventionally grown foods find that organic foods are more nutritious, sometimes significantly so. A study conducted by Theo Clark, a chemistry professor at Truman State University in Missouri found that organic oranges contained 30 percent more vitamin C than conventionally grown oranges even though they were only about one-half the size. Similar results were found in a 2001 report published by the Soil Association, the leading organic farming organization in the United Kingdom. The report titled, "Organic Farming, Food Quality and Human Health," found that organic crops are higher in vitamin C, essential minerals, and phytonutrients, which are compounds that protect plants from disease and pests and are known to be beneficial in treating cancer. Shane Heaton, a nutritionist, compiled the report after examining over 400 published papers that compared organic and conventional foods in terms of food safety, and nutritional content. In a similar published study, nutrition specialist Virginia Worthington surveyed forty-one published studies comparing the nutrient content of organic and conventional crops. She found that organic crops contain 27 percent more vitamin C, 21.1 percent more iron, 29.3 percent more magnesium, and 13.6 percent more phosphorus, and 15.1 percent less nitrates than conventional crops. A study by food scientists at the University of California, Davis, and published in the *Journal of Agricultural and Food Chemistry*, found that organic corn had 52 percent more vitamin C than conventional corn. The study also found that marionberries raised using organic and sustainable farming methods contain significantly higher levels of polyphenols, which are cancer-fighting antioxidants, than conventionally grown foods. Researchers in Italy found that organic peaches and pears also contained higher levels of polyphenols, as well as more ascorbic acid.

Improved Soils, Less Energy, Higher Profits

The benefits of organic agriculture extend to farmers and

the environment. A twenty-one-year study conducted in Switzerland and published in the journal *Science* found that while organic crop yields averaged 20 percent less than conventional crop yields, this was more than compensated by a 50 percent reduction in energy and fertilizer, 97 percent reduction in pesticides, and soils richer in nutrients. Researchers concluded that organic farming used resources more efficiently and was a viable alternative to conventional farming.

Critics of organic farming say it cannot match yields produced by conventional agriculture. However, a study funded by the USDA and published in the journal *Nature* refuted that claim. Researchers at Washington State University compared conventional and organic apple production in Washington over a six-year period and found that the organic system produced better soil quality, comparable yields to conventional, higher profits, greater energy efficiency, and firmer, better-tasting apples. A ten-year study conducted by researchers at the University of Minnesota found that net returns on organic corn and soybeans were comparable to those produced using conventional methods, without taking the organic price premium into account. A 1999 study conducted at Iowa State University found that organic soybean farmers earned a profit of $482.30 per acre compared with $91.02 earned by conventional soybean farmers.

A twenty-three-year study conducted by the Rodale Institute found that organic soils can help mitigate global warming. Through a process called carbon sequestration, organic soils act as "sinks" to capture atmospheric carbon dioxide, which is responsible for 80 percent of global warming, and convert it into useful carbon that helps stimulate plant growth. According to Rodale, converting 10,000 medium-sized farms in the United States to organic production would be equivalent to taking 1,174,400 cars off the road in terms of capturing carbon dioxide in the soil.

Organic Valley's Ripple of Benefits

Organic Valley, the nation's largest organic farming cooperative, based in LaFarge, Wisconsin, offers an excellent example of how organic farming can produce a positive impact from the soil to human health and society. Consumers benefit by purchasing more than 4 million gallons of the cooperative's wholesome organic milk each year. Organic Valley's 650 farmers benefit by earning nearly double what they would earn for producing conventional milk, which, in turn, saves family farms. In 2002, Organic Valley brought 94 farmers into the cooperative and added 15,000 acres to organic production nationwide, which also helped preserve soil and water resources. Finally, rural communities benefit because Organic Valley contracts with many small rural dairy processing facilities nationwide that otherwise may have gone out of business and lost jobs.

George Siemon, chief executive officer of Organic Valley says this "ripple" of benefits is a measure of the cooperative's success. "We look at how many farms we've been able to save, how many acres of land we've gotten into the organic system, and how many jobs we are supporting in rural communities," he says.

Chapter 8

GOT LOCAL ORGANIC MILK?

At first glance, Francis Thicke's 236-acre dairy farm in rural Iowa looks similar to neighboring farms. There are rolling green hills, a big farmhouse, and even a big red barnlike building. However, a closer look reveals a completely different system of agriculture, one that offers a promising model of organic production that serves and is supported by a local economy.

Thicke's farm, called Radiance Dairy, is certified organic. Compared to large-scale conventional dairies, Radiance is tiny with sixty-five cows that produce about 2,000 gallons of milk each week. Every drop is organic along with its yogurt, cheeses, and soft ice cream mix.

Radiance Dairy reflects a growing national appetite for organic dairy products. During the 1990s, sales of organic dairy products increased 500 percent. Maine leads the nation with more than 10 percent of the state's dairies, 50 of 420, now producing organic milk. The nation's two largest organic dairy producers are Organic Valley, based in LaFarge, Wisconsin, and Horizon Organic Dairy, based in Boulder, Colorado. Both sell milk nationally, unlike Radiance, which refuses to sell even regionally. More about that later.

Different Philosophies and Methods

About the only thing Radiance has in common with conventional dairies is that both raise cows and produce milk. Beyond that the two approaches diverge in philosophy and method. In the conventional-industrial system, the emphasis is on production. Cows are raised as milking machines, given hormones to boost milk production, and confined in high-tech, large-scale dairy operations. In contrast, smaller organic operations, such as Radiance, aim to raise healthy crops and animals that will naturally produce more nutritious foods. Cows are fed organic grasses and grains, given ample space to graze outdoors, and treated more humanely.

The differences between the two systems begin with the cows. While most conventional dairies raise the familiar black and white Holsteins, Thicke breeds the smaller, brown Jerseys. "Holsteins produce more milk, but Jersey cow milk contains higher butterfat, lactose, protein, and minerals," he says.

In conventional dairies, cows are confined in a feedlot or barn and given limited access to outdoors. In contrast, organic dairy production requires that cows have freedom of movement and access to outdoor pasture for grazing.

Thicke grazes his cows in pastures called "paddocks" twice a day after milking. His land is divided into 60 paddocks and over time he rotates the cows through all the paddocks so that they receive fresh, nutritious grass every time in the field. Thicke says this "controlled grazing" system enhances cows' health by giving them exercise outdoors as opposed to being confined.

The grazing system is also more energy efficient than

confinement. In conventional dairy operations, forage is harvested, chopped, put in storage bins, and brought to the confined cows. The manure is then collected and hauled out to pasture. Radiance does the opposite. "All we do is open the gate and let the cows go out to pasture where they eat and spread their manure, which enriches the soil," he says. "We save labor and energy with a well-designed pasture system."

Humane Treatment

Thicke believes cows are meant to eat primarily forages, not grains, such as corn, that are fed to cows at conventional dairies. Radiance cows eat grasses, chicory, clover, and alfalfa, along with some barley and soybeans for protein. All feeds are organic, which is required for organic certification.

Thicke has stopped using corn as feed because of the increasing concerns about contamination from genetically engineered corn grown in the area. He sees problems with transgenic crops. "I think they will fail because we don't have a deep enough knowledge about DNA in an ecological context," he says. Thicke sees similar problems with GE bovine growth hormone (rBGH) that conventional cows receive to increase milk production. He states, "rBGH pushes cows' metabolic systems outside of their normal range, aside from how it could hurt human health."

Organic certification requires humane treatment of animals, and Radiance Dairy cows receive plenty of it. In addition to access to fresh air and sunshine and a nutritious organic diet, the cows are not given antibiotics or feeds that increase production. "We don't push for higher production," says Thicke. "The quality of milk is better if you don't push." Conventionally bred cows produce milk for an average of two years; Radiance cows produce milk much longer, sometimes until they are 12 or even 15 years old.

The trend in "high-tech" conventional dairies is robotic milking because it is more "efficient." Thicke sees the need for the soft touch of traditional animal husbandry. "It is important to have direct contact with the animals," he says. "Cows are social animals and like contact with human beings if they are treated well." This is evident when Thicke takes groups from local schools, who often visit Radiance Dairy, out to pasture to see the cows. Some cows will mingle with the students and respond warmly to petting by licking students' clothes or feet.

Importance of Soil Health

Organic agriculture places heavy emphasis on soil health and this is just as important in organic dairy production. "Building soil is critical for good crops and animals," says Thicke, who has a doctoral degree in soil science and worked as a national program leader for soils with the USDA Extension Service prior to owning Radiance.

Before Thicke purchased the farm in 1996, the land had been a typical, conventional Iowa soybean and corn farm. "The soil was pretty beat up," he says. Thicke planted grasses and legumes, such as clover, for grazing and producing hay. These crops also help to enrich the soil and prevent erosion.

The cows contribute to soil improvement by spreading manure on the ground. Thicke also composts manure, which is a common practice among organic farmers. Properly composted manure stabilizes nutrients and kills human pathogens.

Enriching the soil is an ongoing process. "You must have constant input of organic material into the soil to feed soil microbes," says Thicke. "You can't do it just one time and be done."

In addition to improving the soil, Thicke has taken steps to increase plant and wildlife diversity, another goal of organic agriculture. He planted honey locust trees that provide shade for cows in pasture and produce pods that cows will eat as a snack. "Other farmers thought I was crazy to grow them, but they are easy to grow and co-exist well with cows," says Thicke. Letting trees and brush grow on fence lines of his property has increased wildlife habitats and more birds and squirrels have appeared on the land. Little steps like this make a difference. "Properly done organic farming protects natural resources, such as soil, water quality and air," he says.

Thicke's approach to dairy production is the same as that of other organic farmers who nourish the soil to grow healthy and strong crops. He gives the cows everything they need to be healthy and strong, and they in turn produce nutritious milk. It's not a complicated system.

Local Production for Local Consumption

Of 1,000 dairy farms in Iowa, Radiance Dairy is the only one that processes milk on the farm. In a small processing facility, Thicke and his employees use modern equipment to milk the cows, then store, pasteurize, and bottle the milk. Radiance does not homogenize its milk. Thicke believes homogenization reduces the milk's nutritional value.

Radiance whole organic milk looks and tastes richer than conventional milk with a thick layer of cream on top. The lowfat and skim milk also taste richer because of the higher content of protein and milk sugar.

Radiance milk is always fresh from the farm because it is only sold locally at supermarkets and restaurants in Fairfield, Iowa. Demand for Radiance organic milk is strong in this small Iowa town of 10,000, which is unique in that a significant percentage of its population buys organic foods. "We have a good market here," says Thicke, who wants to keep his production local, believing that expanding regionally would bring unwanted challenges. It's not that people don't want him to expand. "We often get calls from people in Des Moines and other areas who want our milk," he says.

Remaining local demonstrates Thicke's commitment to community-supported agriculture (CSA), which aims to reestablish the connection between consumers and farmers that has been severed by modern agriculture. In the United States, food travels an average of 1,300 miles from the farm to the retail shelf. Nearly every state buys up to 90 percent of its food from somewhere else, which causes billions of dollars to leak from state economies each year. CSA helps stem the losses by developing regional food supplies that build local economies. In a CSA program, consumers pay a membership fee to a local farmer and receive fresh organic produce throughout the growing season. CSA establishes a mutually beneficial relationship between farmers and consumers. Farmers gain a ready market and fair compensation for their crops, while consumers receive locally grown organic foods at prices below retail. Money remains in the community. In the process consumers learn how their food is produced, gain a greater appreciation for organic farmers, and often participate in the farming work. In addition, CSA saves energy because no long distance transportation costs are involved. CSA is a growing trend in the United States with more than 1,000 programs nationwide.

Thicke promotes community-based food systems through a Food and Society Policy Fellowship he received from the WK Kellogg Foundation, which is a national program that aims to improve communications about food and agriculture issues in the United States.

While structured differently than a CSA program, Radiance Dairy is essentially the same because it supports Francis Thicke's farm and gives Fairfield consumers a reliable source for fresh, organic milk. "Local production for local consumption," as Thicke likes to say.

Organic Valley's chief executive officer George Siemon says he supports milk producers like Radiance that connect directly with local markets. "We like to get beat out by local competition," he says. Organic Valley produces and sells regional sub-brands, "California Pasture" and "New England Pasture."

Thicke sees CSA as vital for the future of agriculture. "I think we will see a dramatic growth in community-based food systems in coming years," says Thicke. "These will provide fresher, safer, and more secure food supplies for local consumers, protect natural resources, and contribute to the prosperity and renewal of rural communities."

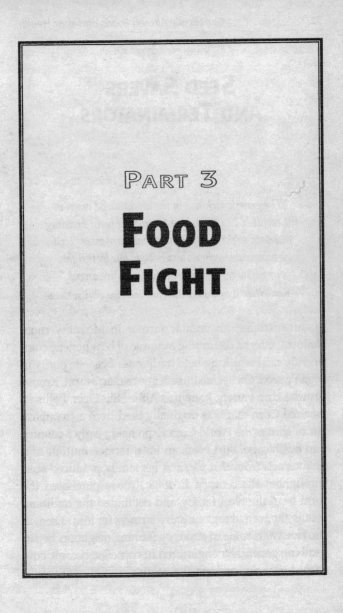

PART 3

FOOD
FIGHT

Chapter 9

SEED SAVERS
AND TERMINATORS

*"The genetic richness of the world's food crops is
the result of 12,000 unbroken years of plant breeding
and seed selection by farmers and gardeners. That
irreplaceable genetic diversity is our birthright,
our heritage, and our legacy. Seeds are sacred."*

—Ken Whealy, executive director, Seed Savers Exchange

Laura Krouse, an organic farmer in Mount Vernon, Iowa, offers a disturbing example of how genetic engineering can break long-held traditions of genetic purity in organic seed. On her small, seventy-two-acre farm, Krouse grows a corn variety, known as Abbe Hills Open Pollinated Seed Corn that was originally bred from a champion ear of corn at the World Corn Expo held nearly a century ago in Chicago. Burt Neal, an Iowa farmer, multiplied a few kernels from that ear, and his family produced seed throughout the century. In 1988 Krouse purchased the farm from the Neal family, and continued the tradition, selling the corn to organic dairy farmers for feed. Then, in the late 1990s some of Krouse's farming neighbors began growing genetically engineered Bt corn. She became concerned that pollen from the neighbor's GE corn would cross-pollinate with her corn and destroy the genetic purity of the heirloom variety. To prevent this, Krause planted the corn in the middle of her field and used the outer rows as a "buffer" to isolate it as far as possible from the GE corn. Despite the precautions, seed from her 2001 crop tested positive for genetically engineered material.

As a result of the contamination, Krouse lost half her business. Even worse was the loss of the corn's genetic purity—in just one season. "Contamination is permanent," says Krouse, who also teaches biology at nearby Cornell College. "The kinds of problems that have hurt me give a preview of the economic and environmental consequences that could happen on a large scale."

Seed Savers

Prior to the contamination, Krouse preserved the purity of her corn by saving seed from each crop. Seed saving is a time-honored tradition practiced by one-half of the world's farmers who uphold an eternal cycle of nature. Farmers plant crops in spring, harvest them in fall, and save seed for the next season's planting. Seed saving helps to maintain genetic diversity and preserve the genetic purity of seed varieties.

About 140 miles north of Laura Krouse's farm lies another farm dedicated to the ancient practice of seed saving, Seed Savers Exchange. Here on 170 acres tucked away amidst the rolling hills of northeast Iowa, Seed Savers preserves a treasure of genetic diversity in the form of heirloom seeds and plants. "Our mission is to increase genetic diversity to people, who are growing healthy foods for their families," says Kent Whealy, who along with his wife Diane are founders and directors of the Seed Savers Exchange.

Seed Savers attracts two things in large numbers: people and seed. SSE has more than 8,000 members, mostly farmers and gardeners in the United States and Canada, who want to preserve the tradition and purity of heirloom vegetables, flowers, and herbs that are often passed down from generation to generation. Members save their seeds and list their offerings each year in Seed Savers' annual 500-page yearbook. For a small fee, members can purchase seeds from other members. In this way, rare seed varieties are preserved.

In addition, Seed Savers maintains a huge collection of seed, 24,000 varieties and growing each year. Whealy and his staff carefully preserve each variety. Seed is cleaned and dried to optimum moisture levels, heat-sealed into foil packets, and then stored in temperature and humidity-controlled rooms. Exposed to the elements some varieties will last only a year, but under Seed Savers' tender care seed life can be extended to forty to fifty years. "Our goal is to keep them really strong for as long as we can," says Whealy.

Seed Savers sells seed to gardeners, growers of specialty organic crops, community supported agriculture programs, and seed companies.

Cornucopia of Diversity

A look at the produce section of an average supermarket and one would think there was one variety of lettuce, Iceberg; one tomato, Beefsteak; one potato, Burbank; and two types of apples: Gold and Red Delicious. A look at

Seed Savers' annual catalog shatters those illusions with a cornucopia of plant diversity. Want tomatoes? Seed Savers' maintains 5,500 varieties. In rich full color the catalog features varieties such as "Cherokee Purple," "German Pink," "Mexico Midget," and "White Beauty," to name a few. Seed Savers' other large collections include 5,200 varieties of beans, 2,000 of pepper, 1,200 of pea, and 1,000 of lettuce. In its orchard, Seed Savers shows there is more to apples than Gold and Red Delicious by growing 700 hundred varieties. According to Whealy, 7,000 apple varieties existed at one time.

Many vegetable seed varieties maintained by Seed Savers were originally brought to North America by European immigrants; others were grown by Native Americans, Mennonites, and Amish. Seed Savers also funded seed-collecting expeditions to Eastern Europe and Russia to preserve about 4,000 vegetable varieties.

Seed Savers also maintains 600 corn varieties, and Whealy wants to preserve them from the genetic drift problems experienced by Laura Krouse. Seed Savers purchased 700 acres from a nearby farm where corn varieties will be grown. "We will plant isolation gardens to protect corn," says Whealy.

He sees genetic engineering as a threat to plant diversity. "The agricultural biotech industry is currently doing everything possible to genetically and legally prevent the saving of seed," says Whealy.

Control of Seed

While Seed Savers views seed as a heritage to be saved and shared, biotechnology companies view it as "intellectual property" to be protected with patents, lawsuits, if necessary, and technologies that render it sterile.

Over the last century, seed and biotechnology companies have gained increasing control over seed through two strategies. One strategy was the development of hybrid plant varieties. This involved breeding two plant lines from different genetic backgrounds to produce greater yields. However, seeds produced from hybrids were not as productive as the parent seed, which forced farmers to purchase new seed each year. The second strategy was lobbying the government to establish laws controlling the sale and distribution of seed. This culminated in 1985 when the United States Patent and Trademark Office began allowing seed companies to patent seeds in the same way companies and individuals patent unique products or inventions. Armed with patents, seed companies can charge licensing fees to other seed companies for the use of proprietary germ plasm to produce new varieties and to charge farmers "technology fees" for the one-time use of seed varieties. The two strategies delivered a one-two punch to seed saving for many farmers, rendering it impractical with hybrids first and illegal with patents second.

Seeing the profit potential of licensing and selling patented seed, biotechnology companies engaged in a buying frenzy of seed companies in the late 1990s. Monsanto spent an estimated $9 billion to buy eight seed companies and became the second largest seed company in the world. DuPont purchased Pioneer Hi-Bred International, which is the world's largest seed company. Novartis, which was the product of a merger between two large

Swiss companies, merged with Zeneca to form Syngenta, the third largest seed company. Dow Chemical purchased two large U.S. seed companies and three in Brazil. As a result of the mergers, the top ten seed companies in the world controlled about 30 percent of the $23 billion commercial seed markets.

Lawsuits against Farmers

To protect their patents on genetically engineered seed, biotechnology companies will sue farmers suspected of "patent infringement." The most famous case involved a Canadian farmer, Percy Schmeiser, who Monsanto sued for growing GE herbicide resistant canola without paying the annual licensing fee. Schmeiser argued that his crop was cross-pollinated from a neighboring field or that seed blew onto his field from a passing truck. Monsanto argued that 90 percent of the field contained GE canola, which was too much to be caused by pollen drift. Judges in the case and in subsequent appeals ruled in Monsanto's favor. The controversial decision angered many farmers because the judge in the case ruled that a farmer is responsible for patented genes in his crop, *no matter how they got there.* Commenting on the absurdity of the decision, an editorial in the *Minneapolis Star Tribune* stated, "It's like making the Alaskans pay Exxon for the oil they collected in Prince William Sound."

Monsanto has initiated similar patent infringement lawsuits against many U.S. farmers. The company hires private investigators to check on farmers suspected of saving or growing GE seed illegally. Some farmers have fought back, saying they have a right to save seed.

Terminator

The latest and most controversial strategy developed by seed companies to control seed is a genetic engineering technology that makes seed sterile. The technology, dubbed "Terminator" by GE activists, was developed in the late 1990s by Delta and Pine Land, the largest cottonseed company in the United States, in collaboration with the USDA. Scientists genetically engineered seeds with a gene complex that forces the resulting plants to produce sterile seeds. The patented "Technology Protection System," as it was originally named, aimed to protect the intellectual property of both GE and non-GE plants, making seed saving impossible and forcing farmers to buy new seed each year. Scientists also hoped the technology would block GE genes from escaping into the environment and cross-pollinating with weeds and other crops. News of the Terminator created a furor among environmentalists and farmers who saw the technology as another instrument for corporate control of seed and as a threat to the environment due to Terminator genes that could spread to other plants causing sterility. As a result of the backlash, Terminator technology has not been commercialized. However, development and patenting of Terminator technology quietly continues.

To those who view seed as sacred, Terminator technology is criminal. "From our perspective, trying to keep all this seed material alive and preserving genetic richness, it is just immoral to have biotech companies kill seed," says Kent Whealy.

Chapter 10

THE BATTLE OVER GE WHEAT

"This is a fundamental problem. The development of genetically engineered wheat shouldn't occur because our customers don't want it."

—Todd Leake, wheat farmer from Emerado, North Dakota

Stephen Jones is a lone crusader fighting to defend a venerable American tradition: the land-grant university system, which was established in 1862 to provide higher education to common citizens who were denied access to elite universities. Research and extension services at the universities aimed to serve the public interests, those of farmers and consumers. Today, Jones, a wheat breeder at Washington State University, says land-grant institutions increasingly serve the interests of corporations, particularly biotechnology companies.

A case in point is that most land-grant universities conducting wheat research are developing varieties that contain Monsanto's genetically engineered Roundup Ready gene. Is this serving the public good? Jones doesn't think so. "Monsanto doesn't have a wheat breeding program. They have to release Roundup Ready wheat through the land-grant universities," he says. Monsanto has established partnerships with land-grant universities who receive funding to develop GE wheat.

Varieties Given Freely

Jones's wheat-breeding program may be the only one among U.S. land-grant universities that is non-GE and has no financial ties to corporations. His research focuses on traditional non-GE winter wheat, as well as perennial and organic wheat. Jones continues a wheat-breeding program founded in 1894 that has developed many varieties that have benefitted farmers and consumers. Every variety was given to farmers for free. "Wheat comes out of land-grant universities and is owned by farmers," says Jones.

In the new world of biotechnology, with its patents on GE seeds, that tradition will end. When Monsanto's Roundup Ready GE wheat is introduced, farmers will pay a licensing fee and be forbidden from saving the seed, an arrangement Jones describes as "renting the seed." "The owner of the seed is the person who grows it," he says. How could someone own the 30,000 genes in wheat?"

Controversy Over GE Wheat

Control over wheat is looming as the next and perhaps most important battleground in the controversy over GE crops. After introducing GE varieties for the two main field crops, corn and soybean, Monsanto targeted number three, wheat, which is grown extensively in North Dakota, Montana, and Washington and in the Canadian province of Saskatchewan. Like its corn and soy counterparts, Roundup Ready wheat is "ready" to be doused with sprays of the company's Roundup herbicide and not die, unlike the weeds. The company aims to start selling seed to farmers in Canada and the United States by 2005 based on market acceptance.

Unlike GE corn and soy, which are processed to make ingredients, wheat is more closely associated with finished foods, such as bread, cereals, and baked goods. Hence, there is more concern that consumers will react negatively to genetic manipulation of their daily bread.

Wheat buyers in Europe, Asia, and the Middle East reacted to Monsanto's plans with a big thumbs down. A 2002 survey conducted by U.S. Wheat Associates, an industry trade group, found "an overwhelming rejection" of GE wheat among Asian buyers, millers, and users. The European Millers Association says its members will stop buying North American wheat if farmers in the United States and Canada grow it. A study by Robert Wisner, a grain market economist at Iowa State University, predicts that the introduction of GE wheat would result in a loss of 30 to 50 percent of United States' wheat exports.

Despite the negative reaction, Monsanto plans to forge ahead, saying it will segregate transgenic wheat from conventional. The company is conducting secret field trials in United States' wheat-producing states and Canadian provinces. The reaction among farmers and wheat exporters has also been negative. A coalition of United States' farm groups filed a petition asking the agricultural department to stop development of GE wheat until its environmental and economic impacts can be assessed. In Canada, a survey by the University of Manitoba found that nearly 90 percent of farmers would not grow GE wheat. The Canadian Wheat Board asked Monsanto to withdraw its application for commercial approval of GE wheat because of imminent rejection by export buyers.

Market rejection would devastate farmers in wheat-growing regions. North Dakota produces an estimated 55 percent of all the hard, red spring wheat grown in the United States each year, which is valued at $1 billion annually. Montana's crop is worth about one-half that. Both states rely heavily on exports.

Sarah Vogel, an attorney and former North Dakota Agriculture Commissioner, questions the intelligence of growing GM wheat. "Eighty percent of customers don't want it. What is the point of raising it?"

With such high stakes, lawmakers in North Dakota and Montana have proposed bills that would limit the introduction of GE wheat or assign liability for contamination of non-GE or organic wheat. No legislation has passed due to lobbying by Monsanto. In North Dakota, Monsanto threatened to pull its research funding from the state's land-grant university.

Ancient Grain, Modern Threat

"Every Japanese wheat buyer who has visited Montana has said, 'we don't want GE wheat,'" says Bob Quinn, an organic farmer in Montana.

Quinn offers an excellent example of organic farming's innovative nature. In 1977, Quinn, who has a Ph.D. in plant biochemistry, obtained seed from an ancient Egyptian wheat variety and, perceiving the grain's value, propagated it. The seed spawned a new organic market, trademarked under the "kamut" name, which is the ancient Egyptian term for wheat. The USDA recognizes kamut as a protected variety that can only be grown organically. Quinn and several other farmers produce organic kamut on more than 4,000 acres in Montana.

Today, Quinn's ancient grain faces a modern threat in GE wheat. He is working with scientists at Montana State University to determine the risk of cross-pollination from GE wheat and developing a quality control program to prevent contamination. "The more guarantees we have for segregation, the better," says Quinn.

Quinn and other organic farmers have reason to fear contamination. Research by Anita Brule-Babel, a plant geneticist at the University of Manitoba in Winnipeg, found that the release of Roundup Ready wheat would be environmentally unsafe because the GE wheat would rapidly pass its herbicide-resistant genes onto weeds, making them stronger. Moreover, the study found that even small amounts of pollen flow from GE wheat will lead to high levels of genetic contamination of non-GE wheat. "Zero tolerance will not be possible when GE crops are released," says Brule-Babel.

Battle of Saskatchewan

In Saskatchewan, organic farmers are taking legal action to stop GE wheat after losing their market for organic canola due to GE contamination. For many years, the provinces's organic farmers relied on canola to control weeds and maintain soil fertility as part of their crop rotations. They also earned a combined $200,000 per year selling canola to export markets, such as Europe. Those days are gone. Saskatchewan's organic farmers don't grow canola anymore because GE canola has become so widespread that it has contaminated the entire crop. "With the proliferation of GE canola it is almost impossible to buy uncontaminated seed let alone contend with contamination from pollen drift," says Arnold Taylor, an organic farmer who is also president of the Saskatchewan Organic Directorate, an organic farmers group.

As a result, the province's organic farmers launched a class-action lawsuit against Monsanto and Aventis in 2002. The farmers claim damages from GE contamination have cost them their entire European market for organic canola, amounting to an estimated $14 million in losses.

The farmers want an injunction to stop the introduction of GE wheat. After losing canola because of contamination, the farmers are drawing a line on GE wheat. "Wheat is more important than canola," says Marc Loiselle, an organic farmer and communications director for the Saskatchewan Organic Directorate. "It's the last remaining major crop in North America that is not genetically engineered, and we have to protect the integrity of organic farming in Saskatchewan."

A lawsuit document states that the introduction of GE wheat ". . . will also cause the decline if not the demise of the Saskatchewan organic industry." Taylor says, "We have to do this to protect our position in the marketplace."

The lawsuit is the first of its kind launched by organic farmers against biotechnology companies. Taylor says it could set a precedent for future legal actions. "This is a pivotal case that's getting worldwide interest," he says. "It's important that we win because it will set a precedent in most jurisdictions. If we win, it will have worldwide impact."

Chapter 11

ORGANIC
AT RISK

*"This is a life and death struggle for your industry.
Genes are crossing now, and your products are
becoming contaminated. You won't have a market
in the next five years."*

—Jeremy Rifkin, founder and president,
The Foundation on Economic Trends (from a
presentation given at Natural Products Expo East
trade show in Washington, D.C., October 2002)

Few topics raise the ire of Michael Potter more than genetic engineering. Potter, founder and president of Eden Foods, an organic food manufacturer based in Clinton, Michigan, says genetic engineering is "an affront to organic agriculture and the most serious threat to the freedom of humanity from corporate exploitation ever."

Potter is angry because he and other organic food manufacturers must deal with the growing threat that genetically modified organisms (GMO) will contaminate their products causing expensive product recalls and the loss of organic certification and even their businesses.

GE contamination causes problems for others who value organic foods. For consumers, contamination can destroy their faith in organic as the one food type that provides a haven from the risks of genetic engineering. For organic farmers, contamination can ruin the sale of a crop and cause the loss of organic certification, threatening their livelihood.

Pollen Problems

The National Organic Program, which sets standards for production of organic foods, prohibits the use of genetic engineering in organic production. Unfortunately, GE genes end up in places where they shouldn't be—such as David Vetter's organic corn. Vetter, an organic farmer in Marquette, Nebraska, has seen his corn crop contaminated by GE corn in each of the last three growing seasons. "We haven't found anything that doesn't have some levels (of genetically engineered material)," he says.

The problem is that corn is a prolific pollinator: each plant sheds millions of pollen grains into the air. Pollen, which comes from the male tassel, travels by wind or insects to other corn plants where it comes into contact with the silk produced by the "female" ear shoot of the plant. Through this cross-pollination, pollen passes its genes from GE to organic corn.

As a responsible organic farmer, Vetter does all he can to prevent GE contamination. He plants as far away from his neighbors' GE corn as possible and he plants later so that their corn pollinates before his does. He uses plants as buffer strips and evergreen trees to block pollen flow. Despite the precautions, his corn has tested positive for GMOs though at very low levels, below 0.1 percent.

"Tip of the Iceberg"

With GE corn accounting for more than 30 percent of all corn grown in the United States, GE contamination is increasingly a problem for organic and conventional farmers. For example, GE StarLink corn, grown mainly in Iowa and Nebraska, was on just 1 percent of corn acreage in the United States in 2000, yet it contaminated as much as 25 percent of the total corn harvest.

Contamination is also a problem in soybeans although soy plants do not cross-pollinate. With soybeans, contamination is more likely to occur during the grain-handling process, ranging from the farmers' fields to grain elevators and food-manufacturing facilities. During this process, GE soybeans can mix with non-GE and organic soy. Such commingling often occurs because the grain-handling system is designed to move commodity crops such as corn and soybeans en masse, not to create separate streams of GE and non-GE grains.

Seed contamination is another problem. The challenges of producing uncontaminated corn seed in the United States forced one organic seed company, Great Harvest Organics, to move its production to Argentina. Contamination is so widespread in corn that many agricultural experts believe it is now impossible to find genetically pure seed. The problem also affects soybean seed. In 2002, GMOs were detected in foundation soybean seed produced at North Dakota State University. The discovery was disturbing because the contamination struck the very basis of seed production, foundation varieties, which are bred by agricultural universities to be genetically pure.

A nationwide survey conducted by the Organic Farming Research Foundation found that contamination from GE crops is causing increasing economic and operational hardships for organic farmers. According to the survey, 8 percent of respondents indicated that their organic farm operation has borne some direct costs or damages related to the presence of GMOs. Nearly half, 46 percent, rated the risk of exposure and possible GE contamination of their organic farm products as moderate or great. OFRF executive director Bob Scowcroft says the problem may just be "the tip of the iceberg."

Identity Preservation

To avoid contamination, Eden Foods and other organic food manufacturers must use a system of identity preservation (IP), which aims to preserve the non-GE and organic integrity of crops and food products through all stages of production—from the farm to the store shelf. IP requires strict growing and handling procedures, including crop segregation, field inspections, equipment cleaning, sampling, and GMO testing.

Eden contracts with several hundred organic farmers to grow soybeans that are used to make the company's flagship product, Edensoy soymilk.

"We have to find growers who are willing to take a risk and grow non-GE crops," says Potter.

According to terms of the contract, Eden will not buy crops that test positive for GMOs. The farmers grow foundation seed varieties supplied by Iowa State University's food grade soybean breeding program that are grown specifically to exclude GMOs.

fair," says Potter. "If I'm damaged who pays
ganic community does and not the industry
ment. It's ludicrous."

phens, president of Nature's Path Foods, an
l manufacturer based in British Columbia,
rganic industry needs to be more proactive.
industry has taken defensive stance on this
s. "We have to take a stronger, more attack-

ogy companies have fought legislation that
liability for GE contamination. Wills says
s need to consider the impact that their
on organic farmers and manufacturers. "I
o basic principles of responsibility and
" he says. "The biotechnology industry is
onsibly with regard to this."

stion

lysis, most organic experts don't believe
veen GE and organic is possible given the
. "Nature is hard-wired to disperse its
s," says Fred Kirschenmann, executive
eopold Center for Sustainable Agricul-
me that we even consider it a possibility
rol gene flow."

Kirschenmann, coexistence is secondary
stion of which system of agriculture can
mounting ecological and health crisis
cal-intensive farming methods. "What
y will address this problem?" he asks.
eering is not the answer because it is

Farmers must take steps to prevent accidental GE contamination, such as cleaning harvesting equipment, storage bins, and trucks used to transport soybeans to Eden's facility.

Extensive GMO Testing

Eden conducts extensive tests of soybeans to detect GMOs. One test is a simple dipstick test, similar to a home pregnancy test, that detects the genetically engineered protein. The second test, called polymerase chain reaction (PCR), is performed in a laboratory. Genetic ID, an Iowa-based laboratory, tests Eden's soy. Like a word search on a computer, PCR scans through a sample's DNA to locate genetically engineered genes. When a GE gene is located, the PCR equipment multiplies the targeted gene billions of times until it can be measured precisely. PCR has the ability to detect and quantify the presence of GE gene sequences down to 0.1 percent. Eden Foods rejects soybeans that test above this threshold.

However, identity preservation requires extra time and costs. "It puts an enormous burden on companies like ours to acquire nongenetically polluted organic food," says Potter. "It's ironic how much money we have to spend to supply our customers with what they want."

GMO tests can be expensive. One PCR test can cost $300 or more. David Vetter estimates he has spent $1,500 to test a corn crop worth $4,000.

Low Contamination

GE contamination of organic foods is negligible to date, according to John Fagan, chief executive officer at Genetic

ID. "You can find traces of GMOs in some organic products, but the levels are low, especially compared to conventional food products," he says.

Genetic ID tests many organic corn and soy food products and finds contamination at 0.1 percent or lower, while contamination of foods with conventional corn or soy ingredients can be as high as 50 percent.

The question remains whether organic farmers and manufacturers can keep contamination to a minimum, especially when GE crop acreage continues to grow. For now, Fagan believes the organic industry is keeping the problem under control. "There may be traces, but organic provides a real haven from genetically engineered products," he says.

Another Threat

In addition to contamination, the widespread planting of GE Bt crops threatens to eliminate a favored pest management tool of organic farmers. For many years, these farmers have used a spray containing the naturally occurring Bt bacterium to kill pests. The spray is nontoxic to mammals and does not leave poisonous residues. Now, as more GE Bt crops are grown, insects may develop resistance to Bt, which would render the Bt spray ineffective.

Coexistence or Collision?

Can organic crops coexist next to genetically engineered crops? Organic proponents have doubts. "It depends on what you mean by coexistence. If someone sits next to you in a restaurant and smokes through your whole din-

ner, did you coexist?" s
farmer and bureau chief
Iowa Department of Agri

"We are living up to o
neighbor is polluting u
that?" asks Organic Vall

Organic and biotec
incompatible. While or
that save genetically er
and get sued by biot
favors single-crop, mo
tory farms; organic far
a variety of crops gro
allows a few multin
seed and food sup
growth of local food
nity-supported agric

Proponents of th
collaborating. Orga
etic engineering. Bio
research in organi
can't make any m
farming allows far
out depending o
the chemical ferti
companies.

Accountability

One major issue
biotech to coexis
due to GE conta

tence, let's b
for it? The o
or the gover

Arran Ste
organic cerea
believes the o
"The organic
issue," he say
ing position."

Biotechnol
would assign
the companies
products have
comes down
accountability,
not acting resp

The Big Que

In the final ana
coexistence betw
laws of biology
seeds and gene
director of the
ture. "It amazes
that we can con

According to
to the urgent que
best solve the
caused by chem
kind of technolog

Genetic engi

another technology "fix" that does not address the underlying problems of pest and disease, and worse, it creates more problems.

What's needed, says Kirschenmann, is to understand why problems emerge and to enhance the inherent strengths within ecosystems to address the bases of the problems. This is the time-tested approach of organic agriculture, which aims to strengthen soils, creating healthy plants that can ward off pests and disease.

Kirschenmann believes genetic research can benefit agriculture, not by creating GE crops, but by helping farmers understand how systems function so they can better utilize the strengths inherent in natural ecosystems.

"One thing seems certain," says Kirschenmann. "If we continue to insist on using technologies in accordance with old paradigms that seem unlikely to meet the challenges of the future, they will fail us."

Chapter 12

SEVEN ACTION STEPS
FOR CONSUMERS

*"This debate is long overdue, important, and ultimately,
should be constructive. There are profound differences
between the principles driving today's GE applications
in agriculture versus the principles of organic farming.
The sooner the public understands these differences and
decides which set of principles should shape their food
future, the sooner the country can progress toward more
coherent national food, farm, and technology policies."*

—Charles M. Benbrook, agricultural economist and former
executive of the board on agriculture at the National
Academy of Sciences. (from a presentation given at the
EcoFarm Conference, Monterey, California, January 24, 2003)

More than fifty years ago, a few farsighted individuals
saw the damage being wrought by industrial agriculture with its over-reliance on chemical pesticides and
fertilizers. These pioneering individuals developed a new
system of agriculture, rooted in effective, age-old methods that emphasize the health of soils and plants.

As time passed more farmers began to realize the wis-
dom and practicality of organic agriculture and made the
transition from industrial methods. In the process they

rediscovered farming and became excited about its possibilities. At the same time, many consumers discovered the benefits of organic food. They believe it tastes better, improves their health, preserves the environment, and supports hard-working farmers. This mutually beneficial relationship between farmers and consumers has spurred the growth of the organic food industry.

Organic is more than a trend; it is a movement based on principles of good health, environmental stewardship, and support for farmers and rural communities.

At the same time, there is a countertrend. As the environmental and health problems resulting from over-reliance on agricultural chemicals have become more obvious, the chemical manufacturers needed to find another solution, one that would maintain their dominant position in agriculture. That solution was genetic engineering. With vast scientific, financial, and political resources at their disposal, the multinational chemical companies morphed into biotechnology companies and developed genetically engineered crops. In just a few years these crops have been planted on millions of acres of American farmland and entered the food supply without public knowledge—leaving many unanswered questions about their impact on human health and the environment. Even more disturbing, virtually no safety tests are conducted on the long-term effects of GE foods, which makes every consumer of GMOs a guinea pig in a mass-feeding experiment.

Organic food production offers a better, more sustainable solution to the crisis of modern agriculture than genetic engineering. Organic agriculture has proven to be a viable, economical, and environmentally sound way to produce healthy and safe food. On the other hand, the jury remains out on genetic engineering, which is the latest "silver bullet" of industrial agriculture, taking its tradition of manipulating and dominating nature to a potentially greater level of destruction.

One essential criterion for a beneficial technology, particularly for producing food, is that it "does no harm." Genetic engineering has not met this criterion. Because it manipulates the building block of life, the DNA, genetic engineering is a powerful and unpredictable technology that poses many risks. Studies showing GE crops killing monarch butterflies, threats of new food allergies, evidence of passing on GE genes to weeds, and incidents of GE contamination causing economic damage to farmers are a few examples that cast doubt on genetic engineering's ability to do no harm. On the other hand, increasing evidence shows that organic foods reduce pesticide levels in foods and contain higher levels of nutrients, such as vitamin C and essential minerals. Organic production prevents topsoil erosion, improves soil fertility, protects groundwater, and conserves energy. Organic agriculture offers renewed opportunities for farmers to earn a better, healthier living, which helps revitalize rural communities.

Unfortunately, organic agriculture faces perilous threats from contamination by GE crops and from biotechnology companies that refuse to assume responsibility for their wayward genes. Organic agriculture also faces threats from corporate/government interests that seek to weaken its standards and the integrity of organic food.

Ultimately, consumers may decide which system of

food production prevails, genetic engineering or organic. The war may be waged in corporate boardrooms and on farmers' fields, but it will be decided on the dinner tables of American consumers. "In a democracy like ours people can make up their own minds," says Margaret Mellon of the Union of Concerned Scientists, "They can vote with their forks."

Think Globally, Eat Locally

In addition to voting with their forks, consumers can take positive steps to avoid unlabeled GE foods, eat healthier, stay informed, and become involved in the GE food debate.

SEVEN ACTION STEPS FOR CONSUMERS

1. Avoid Genetically Engineered Foods

This is not easy. Up to 75 percent of processed foods found in retail stores and restaurants contain ingredients derived from GE crops, mainly corn and soybeans. Corn is processed to make flour, starches, oil, and syrup sweeteners. These are found in hundreds of food products, including soda, candies, chips, ice cream, cookies, salad dressings, breads, cereals, margarine, and others. Soybeans are used to make flour, oil, lecithin, protein, and concentrates. These are found in many of the same products listed above and also in soy cheeses, soy sauce, crackers, frozen yogurt, protein powder, tofu dogs, veggie burgers, and others. In general, the less processed packaged foods you eat, the more likely you will be to avoid GE foods.

The two other main GE crops, canola and cotton, are processed into oils that are also found in many processed foods.

Other Crops

Several GE varieties of yellow "crookneck" squash have been commercialized but are not widely grown. GE papayas are grown in Hawaii, but they are only sold to consumers there or on the West Coast. Other GE crops earlier approved for production, including potatoes, tomato, flax, radicchio, and sugarbeets are no longer grown.

Dairy

Dairy products, such as milk, buttermilk, butter, sour cream, and yogurt, may be made with milk from cows treated with the GE bovine growth hormone, rBGH. As with foods containing GE ingredients, dairy products from cows given rBGH are not labeled. Often, labels on rBGH-free dairy products will state, "Milk from cows not treated with rBST/rBGH."

Meat and Poultry, Vitamins, and Enzymes

Meat products may be derived from cattle, hogs, and chickens raised on feed that contains GE corn and soybeans. Again, there are no labels to inform consumers about this.

Vitamins including E, B_2, B_6, B_{12}, and C are derived from or produced with the help of GE organisms. Vitamin E is commonly derived from soy, while vitamin C is derived from corn. Unfortunately, little information is available about these products.

GE bacteria and fungi are used to make enzymes that are used as processing aids in food manufacturing. For example, chymosin is an enzyme derived from GE bacteria that is used to make cheeses. Fourteen enzymes derived from GE bacteria or fungi have been developed. These enzymes are usually not present in the final food product; they are destroyed or removed by further processing and cooking. As a result, they are rarely listed on product labels.

Look for Non-GMO Labels

Some natural and organic food manufacturers label their products "non-GMO," "GE-free," or "not genetically engineered" to indicate that products don't contain GE ingredients.

Resources

• Greenpeace has compiled "The True Food Shopping List," an excellent list of food products that contain and do not contain GE ingredients. The list is available at www.truefoodnow.org and is also available in print.

2. Eat Organic

Buying organic foods offers the best assurance against the risks of genetic engineering because GE substances are prohibited in organic production. Consumers can identify organic foods by looking for the small green and white "USDA Organic" label on products. Certified organic products are labeled according to the following levels of organic content:

1. 100 percent organic. Products contain only organically produced ingredients.

2. Organic. Products contain at least 95 percent organically produced ingredients.

3. Made with organic ingredients. Processed products contain at least 70 percent organic ingredients.

4. Some organic ingredients. Processed products that contain less than 70 percent organic ingredients will list the ingredients that are organically produced.

Resources

• The Organic Trade Association (www.ota.com)

3. Buy Locally Grown Foods

There is nothing better than locally produced fresh fruits and vegetables. Buying local supports organic farmers, keeps food dollars in the community, and reconnects consumers with farmers. There are several ways to buy local:

1. *Farmers markets.* According to the USDA, the number of farmers markets increased 79 percent from 1994 to 2002, expanding to 3,100 markets nationwide with some 19,000 farmers selling their crops. Farmers gain a ready market for their crops and consumers get fresh food at prices lower than retail.

Resources

• Visit the USDA's website on farmers markets at www.ams.usda.gov/farmersmarkets/

- Local Harvest at www.local harvest.org is another good resource.

2. *Community supported agriculture (CSA).* In CSA consumers pay a membership fee to a local farmer and receive fresh organic produce throughout the growing season. Like a farmers market, CSA benefits farmers and consumers. In the process consumers learn how their food is produced and often participate in farming. There are more than 1,000 CSA programs nationwide.

Resources

- Visit the USDA's website on community supported agriculture at www.nal.usda.gov/afsic/csa/

4. Grow Your Own

Gardening is a great hobby, nourishing to the body, mind, and soil. You can also participate in urban agriculture projects that are sprouting up nationwide. Urban gardens allow city dwellers to take food production into their own hands and enjoy the benefits of locally grown organic food.

Resources

- *Organic Gardening* is a perennial favorite magazine. Their website is www.organicgardening.com.

- Fairview Gardens is an urban agricultural project in Southern California. Visit their website at www.fairviewgardens.org.

5. Support Labeling of GE Foods

Write to your congressional representatives and ask them to support legislation requiring mandatory safety testing and labeling of GE foods. Also ask them to increase research funding for organic agriculture and to preserve the integrity of organic standards.

Resource

• An excellent resource is *The Campaign to Label GE Foods*. Visit their website at www.thecampaign.org.

6. Create a GE-free Zone in Your Area

This involves persuading farmers in your area to not grow GE crops, lobbying local officials to pass a GE-free resolution prohibiting plantings of GE crops, or launching a ballot initiative that would ask voters to pass a resolution. Groups have passed GE-free resolutions in seventy towns in Vermont and six in Massachusetts, as well as major cities such as Minneapolis, San Francisco, and Austin, Texas. In 2003, organic food supporters in Mendocino County, California, successfully organized a ballot initiative that aims to make the county a GMO-free zone.

Resources

• www.gefreevt.org
• www.mendocinoorganicnetwork.com

7. Stay Informed About GE Food Issues

Many consumers in the United States remain unaware of

GE foods. The biotechnology industry spends $50 million per year in advertising to persuade American consumers about the benefits of transgenic foods, aiming to prevent a repeat of the consumer backlash that occurred in Europe. Such promotion glosses over the risks of genetic engineering with slick advertising and television commercials showing smiling children or wholesome-looking farmers in lush fields of grain. To be really informed about the issue, you need to look beyond the usual media outlets. There are many excellent websites that contain up-to-date information about GE food issues.

Resources

- CropChoice.com (www.cropchoice.com)
- Organic Consumers Association (www.organic consumers.org)
- Union of Concerned Scientists (www.ucsusa.org)
- Mothers for Natural Law (www.safe-food.org)
- Alliance for Bio-Integrity (www.bio-integrity.org)
- GEO-Pie, University of Cornell (www.comm.cornell. edu/gmo/gmo.html)
- *The Non-GMO Source* (www.non-gmosource.com)

REFERENCES

Chapter 1

Biotechnology Industry Organization. "Biotechnology: A Collection of Technologies." www.bio.org/er/technology_collection.asp (accessed January 23, 2003).

Butler, L. J. "The Profitability of rBST on U.S. Dairy Farms." AgBio Forum, University of California–Davis (July 1999): 111–117.

Charles, Daniel. *Lords of the Harvest: Biotech, Big Money, and the Future of Food*. Cambridge, MA: Perseus, 2001.

Cummins, Ronnie and Lilliston, Ben. *Genetically Engineered Food: A Self-Defense Guide for Consumers*. NY: Marlowe, 2000.

Global Status of Commercialized Transgenic Crops: 2003.

Kirschenmann, Frederick, "Expanding the Vision of Sustainable Agriculture." In *For All Generations: Making World Agriculture More Sustainable*. World Sustainable Agriculture Association, 1997, p. 39.

Swientek, Bob. "Back to the Future." *Prepared Foods* (October 2000).

Chapter 2

AgBioWorld. "31 Critical Questions in Agricultural Biotechnology." www.agbioworld.org.

Benbrook, Charles M. "Impacts of Genetically Engineered Crops on Pesticide Use in the United States: The First Eight Years." *AgBioTech InfoNet Technical Paper 6*. (November 2003): 7.

Benbrook, Charles M. "Troubled Times amid Commercial Success for Roundup Ready Soybeans." *AgBioTech InfoNet Technical Paper* (May 2001): 28–29.

Bucchini, Luca and Goldman, Lynn R. "A Snapshot of Federal Research on Food Allergy: Implications for Genetically Modified Food." Pew Initiative on Food and Biotechnology, 2002.

Commoner, Barry. "Unraveling the DNA Myth: The Spurious Foundation of Genetic Engineering." *Harper's Magazine* (February 2002).

Domingo, Jose L. "Health Risks of GM Foods: Many Opinions but Few Data. *Science* 288 (June 9, 2000): 1748.

Duffy, Michael. "Study Shows No Economic Advantage for Iowa Farmers to Plant GMO Crops," *Leopold Letter* 13 (Winter 2002): 1–2.

Elmore, Roger W. "Glyphosate-Resistant Soybean Cultivar Yields Compared with Sister Lines." *Journal of Agronomy* 93 (March–April 2001): 408–412.

Gurian-Sherman, Doug. "Holes in the Biotech Safety Net: FDA Policy Does Not Assure the Safety of Genetically Engineered Foods." Center for Science in the Public Interest, 2002.

Ho, Mae-Wan; Ryan, Angela; and Cummins, Joe. "Cauliflower Mosaic Promoter—A Recipe for Disaster?" *Microbial Ecology in Health and Disease* (1999): 194–197.

Kimbrell, Andrew. "Industrial Agriculture Will Feed the World," Kimbrell, Andrew. *Fatal Harvest: The Tragedy of Industrial Agriculture.* Washington, D.C.: Island, 2002, p. 50.

Nill, Kimball. "Let the Facts Speak for Themselves: The Contribution of Agricultural Crop Biotechnology to American Farming." *AgBioWorld.* www.agbioworld.org.

Chapter 3

Alliance for Bio-Integrity. www.bio-integrity.org/ext-summary.html.

Biotech-Info. "Dr. Elaine Ingham's Testimony before the New Zealand Royal Commission on Genetic Modification-Executive Summary." www.biotech-info.net/EI_testimony_NZ.html.

Druker, Stephen. "How the U.S. Food and Drug Administration Approved Genetically Engineered Foods despite the Deaths One Had Caused and the Warnings of Its Own Scientists about Their Unique Risks." www.bio-integrity.org/ext-summary.html.

Editor. *Nature Biotechnology* 20, No. 6 (June 2002): 527.

Ho, Dr. Mae-Wan. *ISIS Report*. Institute of Science in Society. (November 1, 2003).

Holmes, M. and Ingham, E.R. "Ecological Effects of Genetically Engineered *Klebsiella Planticola* Released into Agricultural Soil with Varying Clay Content." *Applied Soil Ecology*. 3: 394–399.

Lappe, Marc A., E. Britt, Childress, Chandra, and Setchell, Kenneth D.R. "Alterations in Clinically Important Phytoestrogens in Genetically Modified Soybeans." *Journal of Medicinal Food*, vol. 1, No. 4, (1999) pages 241–245.

MacArthur M. "Triple-Resistant Canola Weeds Found." *Western Producer* (February 10, 2000).

Netherwood, Trudy, et al. "Transgenes in Genetically Modified Soya Survive Passage through the Human Small Bowel but Are Completely Degraded in the Colon." United Kingdom Food Standards Agency, 2002.

Obrycki, John, et al. "Registration of Bt Crops." Ag Biotech InfoNet. www.biotech-info.net/obrycki_comments.html.

Wagner, Holly. "Genetically Modified Crops May Pass Helpful Traits to Weeds, Study Finds." Ohio State University. www.osu.edu/units/research/archive/sungene.htm.

Quist, David and Chapela, Ignacio. "Transgenic DNA Introgressed into Traditional Maize Landraces in Oaxaca, Mexico." *Nature* 414 (November 2001): 541–542.

Chapter 4

National Academy of Sciences, January 17, 2003. "Animal Biotechnology: Science Based Concerns." Committee on Defining Science-Based Concerns with Products of Animal Biotechnology, Health and the Environment, National Research Council, 2002.

Chapter 5

Druker, Steven M. "How the U.S. Food and Drug Administration Approved Genetically Engineered Foods despite the Deaths One Had Caused and the Warnings of Its Own Scientists about Their Unique Risks." Alliance for Bio-Integrity. www.bio-integrity.org/ext-summary.html. Lambrecht, Bill. *Dinner at the New Gene Café*. NY: St. Martin's, 2001.

Levy, Allan S., Derby, Brenda, M. "Report on Consumer Focus Groups on Biotechnology." U.S. Food and Drug Administration. (October, 20, 2000). www.cfsan.fda.gov/~comm/biorpt.html.

Statement of Policy: Foods Derived from New Plant Varieties." U.S. Food and Drug Administration. *Federal Register* (May 29, 1992). www.cfsan.fda.gov/~lrd/biotechm.html.

Chapter 6

Delate, Kathleen. "Organic Agriculture." Iowa State University Extension brochure, (May 2002): p. 2.

Editor. "Organic Trend." *Organic Style.* (September–October 2003): 148.

Haumann, Barbara. "Buying for Organic: Considering the Real Costs. *What's News in Organic* Organic Trade Association. (November–December, 2000).

May, Thomas Garvey. "Organic Produce Sees Strong Growth." *Natural Foods Merchandiser* (June 2002): 26.

Pollan, Michael. *The Botany of Desire: A Plant's Eye-View of the World.* NY: Random House, 2001.

Sligh, Michael. "Organic at the Crossroads." In *Fatal Harvest: The Tragedy of Industrial Agriculture.* Washington, D.C.: Island, 2002, p. 341.

Sligh, Michael. "Organic at the Crossroads." In *Fatal Harvest: The Tragedy of Industrial Agriculture.* Washington, D.C.: Island, 2002. p. 345.

Chapter 7

"Agricultural Pesticides: Management Improvements Needed to Further Promote Integrated Pest Management." U.S. General Accounting Office (GAO-01-815, August 2001): p. 4.

Asami, Danny K, et al. "Comparison of the Total Phenolic and Ascorbic Acid Content of Freeze-Dried and Air-Dried Marionberry, Strawberry, and Corn Grown Using Conventional, Organic, and Sustainable Agricultural Practices." *Journal of Agricultural and Food Chemistry* 51 (February 2003): 1237–1241.

Baker, B. P., et al. "Pesticide Residues in Conventional Integrated Pest Management (IPM)-Grown and Organic Foods: Insights from Three US Data Sets." *Food Additives and Contaminants* 19 (May 2002): 427.

Curl, Cynthia L.; Fenske Richard A.; and Elgethun, Kai. "Organophosphorus Pesticide Exposure of Urban and Suburban Pre-School Children with Organic and Conventional Diets." *Environmental Health Perspectives* (Online, October 2002).

Delate, Kathleen. *Organic Agriculture.* Iowa State University Extension brochure, (May 2002): 16.

Editor. "Organic Trend." *Organic Style.* (September–October 2003): 148.

Gil, María I., et al. "Antioxidant Capacities, Phenolic Compounds, Carotenoids, and Vitamin C Contents of Nectarine, Peach, and Plum Cultivars from California." *Journal of Agricultural and Food Chemistry* 50 (August 2002): 4976–4982.

"Key Findings from the Organic Farming, Food Quality, and Human Health Report."

Soil Association. www.soilassociation.org/web/sa/saweb.nsf/library titles/Briefing_Sheets03082001a.

Mäder, Paul, et al. "Soil Fertility and Biodiversity in Organic Farming." *Science* 296 (May 31, 2002): 1694–1697.

Porter, Paul M., et al. "Organic and Other Management Strategies with Two- and Four-Year Crop Rotations in Minnesota." *Agronomy Journal* 95. (March–April 2003): 233–244.

Reganold, John P., et al. "Sustainability of Three Apple Production Systems." *Nature* 410 (April 19, 2001): 926–930.

ScienceDaily. "Research at Great Lakes Meeting Shows More Vitamin C in Organic Oranges Than Conventional Oranges." American Chemical Society News Release.

www.sciencedaily.com/releases/2002/06/020603071017.html.

Shafer, Kristin. "Nowhere to Hide: Persistent Toxic Chemicals in the U.S. Food Supply." *Pesticide Action Network Report.* (March 2000).

Swan, Shanna, et al. "Geographic Differences in Semen Quality of Fertile U.S. Males." *Environmental Health Perspectives* 111, No. 4 (April 2003): 414–420.

Worthington, Virginia. "Nutritional Quality of Organic Versus Conventional Fruits, Vegetables, and Grains." *The Journal of Alternative and Complementary Medicine* 7, No. 2 (2001): 161–173.

Chapter 8

Van En, Roybn, "What is Community Supported Agriculture and How Does It Work?" University of Massachusetts Extension web page. www.umass.edu/umext/csa/about.html.

Chapter 9

Action Group on Erosion, Technology, and Concentration. "Seed Industry Consolidation: Who Owns Whom?" www.etcgroup.org/article. asp?newsid=186.

Chapter 10

Quinn, Robert M. "Kamut: Ancient Grain, New Cereal." *Perspective on New Crops and Uses.* Alexandria, VA: ASHS, 1999.

Chapter 12

Genetically Engineered Organisms Public Education Project website. Cornell University Cooperative Extension. www.comm.cornell.edu/gmo/who.html.

BIBLIOGRAPHY FOR FURTHER READING

Cummins, Ronnie and Ben Lilliston. *Genetically Engineered Food: A Self-Defense Guide for Consumers.* New York: Marlowe, 2000.

Hart, Kathleen. *Eating in the Dark: America's Experiment with Genetically Engineered Food.* New York: Pantheon, 2002.

Kimbrell, Andrew, ed. *Fatal Harvest: The Tragedy of Industrial Agriculture.* Washington, D.C.: Island, 2002.

Lambrecht, Bill. *Dinner at the New Gene Café.* New York: Thomas Dunne /St. Martin's, 2001.

Rifkin, Jeremy. *The Biotech Century: Harnessing the Gene and Remaking the World.* New York: Tarcher/Putnam, 1998.

Smith, Jeffrey. *Seeds of Deception: Exposing Industry and Government Lies about the Safety of the Genetically Engineered Foods You're Eating.* Fairfield, Iowa: Yes, 2003.

Ticciati, Laura and Robin Ticciati, Ph.D. *Genetically Engineered Foods— Are They Safe? You Decide.* New York: McGraw-Hill /Keats, 1998.

INDEX

ABOUT THE
AUTHOR

Ken Roseboro is editor and publisher of *The Non-GMO Source*, a monthly newsletter that helps farmers and food manufacturers respond to the challenges of genetically engineered foods. Ken has written extensively about GE foods for many agricultural and food industry publications, including *Seed World*, *Seed Today*, *World Grain*, *American Food and Ag Exporter*, *Prepared Foods*, *Food Processing*, *Food Quality*, *European Food and Drink Review*, *Natural Products Industry Insider*, and others. He is also a contributing editor to *Natural Foods Merchandiser* and *Grain Journal*.